D1492929

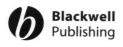
Blackwell
Publishing

Sociology of Health and Illness Monograph Series

Edited by Jonathan Gabe
Department of Social and Political Science
Royal Holloway
Egham
Surrey
TW20 0EX
UK

Current titles:

- **Social Movements in Health (2004),**
  edited by *Phil Brown and Stephen Zavestoski*
- **Health and the Media (2004),**
  edited by *Clive Seale*
- **Partners in Health, Partners in Crime: Exploring the boundaries of criminology and sociology of health and illness (2003),**
  edited by *Stefan Timmermans and Jonathan Gabe*
- **Rationing: Constructed Realities and Professional Practices (2002),**
  edited by *David Hughes and Donald Light*
- **Rethinking the Sociology of Mental Health (2000),**
  edited by *Joan Busfield*
- **Sociological Perspectives on the New Genetics (1999),**
  edited by *Peter Conrad and Jonathan Gabe*
- **The Sociology of Health Inequalities (1998),**
  edited by *Mel Bartley, David Blane and George Davey Smith*
- **The Sociology of Medical Science (1997),**
  edited by *Mary Ann Elston*
- **Health and the Sociology of Emotion (1996),**
  edited by *Veronica James and Jonathan Gabe*
- **Medicine, Health and Risk (1995),**
  edited by *Jonathan Gabe*

Forthcoming titles:

- **The Social Organisation of Healthcare Work (2005),**
  edited by *Davina Allen, Alison Pilnick and Carolyn Wiener*
- **The View From Here: Bioethics and the Social Sciences (2006),**
  edited by *Raymond de Vries, Leigh Turner, Kristina Orfali and Charles Bosk*

Social Movements in Health

Edited by
Phil Brown and Stephen Zavestoski

First published as a special issue of *Sociology of Health and Illness* Volume 26 No 6.

BLACKWELL PUBLISHING
350 Main Street, Malden, MA 02148-5020, USA
108 Cowley Road, Oxford OX4 1JF, UK
550 Swanston Street, Carlton, Victoria 3053, Australia

First published 2005 by Blackwell Publishing Ltd

Library of Congress Cataloging-in-Publication Data has been applied for

ISBN 1-4051-2449-0

A catalogue record for this title is available from the British Library.

Set by Graphicraft Limited, Hong Kong
Printed and bound in the United Kingdom
by TJ International Ltd, Padstow, Cornwall

For further information on
Blackwell Publishing, visit our website:
www.blackwellpublishing.com

Contents

Notes on Contributors

Judith Allsop is a Research Professor in Health Policy at De Montfort University, Leicester. She has written widely on health policy, complaints in health care settings, the health professions and health consumers. Her most recent publications are an edited book: *The Regulation of the Health Professions* with Mike Saks; *Speaking for Patients and Carers: Health Consumer Groups and the Policy Process* with Rob Baggott and Kathryn Jones and, with colleagues, a scoping study on current procedures for the new Council for Health Regulatory Excellence. In the past, she has given advice to various governmental bodies on complaints and has been a member of a Healthcare Commission investigation team. At present she is a member of the investigating committee of the Council for the Regulation of Forensic Practitioners and chairs a lay panel for complaints about health care.

Rob Baggott is Professor of Public Policy and director of the Health Policy Research Unit at De Montfort University, Leicester. His research interests focus on patient and user involvement; public health policy; alcohol policy; health service reform and regulatory politics. Rob's most recent publications include *Public Health: Policy and Policy* (2000) and *Health and Health Care in Britain* (3rd edition, 2004) and *Speaking for Patients and Carers: Health Consumer Groups and the Policy Process* (with Judith Allsop and Kathryn Jones, 2004).

Renée L. Beard is a Doctoral Candidate in the department of Social and Behavioral Sciences at the University of California San Francisco. She will soon complete her PhD on *Managing Memory: Making Alzheimer's patients in clinical practice, advocacy arenas, and everyday life.* She is a Lecturer in Sociology at the University of San Francisco. Her research and teaching interests focus on medical sociology, including lay and expert knowledges, memory, and aging. Recent publications include 'In their voices: identity preservation and the experience of Alzheimer's disease' (2004, *Journal of Aging Studies*, 18.4: 415–428) and 'The Medicalization of Aging' (2002, with C.L. Estes, *Macmillan Encyclopedia of Aging*, 883–886).

Phil Brown is Professor of Sociology and Environmental Studies at Brown University. Since 1999, he has been examining 'contested illnesses' such as asthma, breast cancer and Gulf War-related illnesses, involving public debates over environmental causes and the impact of social movements on those debates. At present he is examining coalitions between environmental organizations and labour unions and other labour organizations. In another project he is studying connections between breast cancer advocacy and environmental justice organizing. He is the author of *No Safe Place: Toxic Waste, Leukemia, and Community Action* (Phil Brown and Edwin Mikkelsen), about the Woburn childhood leukemia cluster. He is editor of *Perspectives in Medical Sociology*, and co-editor of the collection *Illness and the Environment: A Reader in Contested Medicine* (Steve Kroll-Smith, Phil Brown and Valerie Gunter).

Chris Ganchoff is a Ph.D. candidate in Medical Sociology at the University of California, San Francisco. His research interests include the history of biotechnology in California, the relationships between venture capital and life science research, social movements of health and illness and stem cell research. He is currently finishing his research focused on the formation of the California Institute for Regenerative Medicine and the public imagination of stem cell futures.

Melinda Goldner is an Assistant Professor of Sociology at Union College. Her research interests focus on the complementary and alternative medicine (CAM) movement, integrative medicine, online health searches and informal caregiving. Her most recent publications include a chapter on CAM consumers in a book titled *The Mainstreaming of Complementary and Alternative Medicine: Studies in Social Context* (edited by Philip Tovey, Gary Easthope and Jon Adams for Routledge). She also serves as the Associate Book Review Editor for *Complementary Health Practice Review.*

David J. Hess is a Professor in the Department of Science and Technology Studies at Rensselaer Polytechnic Institute. He is the author, editor or coeditor of a dozen books and volumes in the anthropology, history and sociology of science, technology and society. His early work focused on science, health and religious movements, and his more recent work focuses on alternative health movements and sustainability movements. More information and some publications are available at his website at <http://home.earthlink.net/~davidhesshomepage>

Carole Joffe is a Professor of Sociology at the University of California, Davis and a Visiting Professor at the Center for Reproductive Health Policy and Research at the University of California, San Francisco. She is the author of *Doctors of Conscience: The Struggle to Provide Abortion before and after Roe v. Wade*, and *The Regulation of Sexuality: Experiences of Family Planning Workers*. Besides writing for an academic audience, she frequently writes op-eds on reproductive health and reproductive politics for major newspapers. Her current research involves tracking the spread of mifepristone ('RU-486') into various medical settings since FDA approval in 2000. She recently completed two terms as a member of the board of directors of the National Abortion Federation.

Kathryn Jones is a Research Fellow in the Department of Public Policy, De Montfort University, Leicester. Her research interests include user involvement and patients' organisations. A book providing further findings from the study reported here, *Speaking for Patients and Carers: Health Consumer Groups and the Policy Process* with Rob Baggott and Judith Allsop, has recently been published by Palgrave Macmillan.

Maren Klawiter is an Assistant Professor of Sociology in the School of History, Technology and Society, at the Georgia Institute of Technology. She received her Ph.D. in 1999 from the University of California, Berkeley, and from 1999 to 2001 she was a fellow in the Robert Wood Johnson Foundation Scholars in Health Policy Research Program at the University of Michigan. Klawiter's research explores the relationship between subjectivity, social movements and the practices of science, medicine and public health. Her first book, *Reshaping the Contours of Breast Cancer: Disease Regimes, Cultures of Action, and the Bay Area Field of Contention*, is nearing completion. A second book, provisionally entitled *Diagnosing Risk, Prescribing Prevention: Constructing the Breast Cancer Continuum*, explores the pharmaceuticalization of risk in the context of cancer chemoprevention. Her current work focuses on a series of research collaborations between environmental breast cancer activist-experts and university scientists.

Emily S. Kolker is currently a Doctoral Candidate in the Sociology Department at Brandeis University. Her research interests include sociology of the new genetics, medical risk, and gender and health. Her dissertation investigates the intersection between medical genetics, contemporary concepts of risk and kinship relations in families deemed medically at 'high-risk' for hereditary breast and ovarian cancer.

Clare L. Stacey is a Postdoctoral Fellow at the Institute for Health Policy Studies and the Institute for Health and Aging at the University of California, San Francisco. She is currently revising her dissertation into a book on the work identities and labour struggles of home care workers in California. Broad research interests include community based long-term care, low-wage healthcare work and informal/formal caregiving. She is also working with colleagues at UCSF on an ethnographic study of patient stigma in four healthcare organizations.

Tracy Weitz, MPA, is the Associate Director for Public Policy and Community Relations at the University of California, San Francisco (UCSF) National Center of Excellence in Women's Health (CoE) where she develops and refines new models for comprehensive health care for women. She is also the co-Director for the Advancing New Standards in Reproductive Health (ANSIRH) program of the UCSF Center for Reproductive Health Research & Policy, working to expand abortion and other family planning services and training, both nationally and internationally. Ms. Weitz holds a master's degree in public administration with an emphasis in health care, and is currently a doctoral student in Medical Sociology at UCSF.

Stephen Zavestoski is an Assistant Professor of Sociology at the University of San Francisco. His current research examines the role of science in disputes over the environmental causes of unexplained illnesses, and the use of the Internet as a tool for enhancing public participation in federal environmental rulemaking. His work appears in journals such as *Science, Technology and Human Values, Journal of Health and Social Behavior, Social Science & Medicine* and *Sociology of Health and Illness.*

Chapter 1

Social movements in health: an introduction
Phil Brown and Stephen Zavestoski

Health social movements (HSMs) are an important political force concerning health access and quality of care, as well as for broader social change. We define HSMs as collective challenges to medical policy, public health policy and politics, belief systems, research and practice which include an array of formal and informal organisations, supporters, networks of co-operation and media. HSMs make many challenges to political power, professional authority and personal and collective identity. These movements address (a) access to, or provision of, health-care services; (b) disease, illness experience, disability and contested illness; and (c) health inequality and inequity based on race, ethnicity, gender, class and/or sexuality.

This introductory essay has three goals. First, we aim to explain why an entire volume on health social movements is warranted, by specifying the important analytical questions to be answered and by situating the volume in the midst of a growing interest in the topic among scholars from various sociological fields and even other disciplines. Second, we seek to offer an explanation for the phenomenon of health social movements generally, and more specifically what appears to be a recent growth in their presence and power in contemporary societies. We do this by noting the growing tendency across all movements to challenge authority structures, and by emphasising the ways in which HSMs challenge the authority of medicine, science, governments and corporations. Third, we further develop the concept of health social movements, and offer some conceptual tools that may be of use in reading the contributions to the volume, which we introduce in a manner that offers insight into the ways in which they advance our understanding of HSMs.

Why and whence the focus on HSMs?

In the last SHI Monograph, *Health and the Media*, Clive Seale (2003) introduced the volume by pointing to the fact that media studies and the sociology of health and illness 'stand at a distance from one another'. Seale used the Monograph as a vehicle to bridge that gap. The same holds true for health social movements: many medical sociologists have studied such movements without reference to social movement theory and literature, while social movement specialists rarely take up issues of health.

Fortunately, we are seeing recent attention to health social movements that has the potential to reduce this gap. The Society for Social Studies of Science, in both the 2001 and 2003 annual meetings, had a stream of four sessions on the topic. Stemming from that 2003 stream, a special issue of *Science as Culture* on health, the environment, and social movements is now in press, edited by David Hess. The current volume editors were invited to lead a multi-session workshop at the American Sociological Association's Collective Behavior and Social Movements Section Conference in August 2002. A medical social movements symposium was held in Sweden in June 2003, with a resultant special issue of *Social Science and Medicine* on patient-centred movements, edited by Joe Dumit, published in 2004. A special issue on health and the environment of *Annals of the American Academy of Political and Social Science*, in November 2002, focused on the role of health social movements.

Sociology of Health and Illness has published a significant amount of research on health social movements, and it is fitting that this volume reflects this tradition. In our recent article in this journal, Embodied health movements: uncharted territory in social movement research (Brown *et al.* 2004), we put forth our first attempt to systematise the study of these movements. Previous research has focused on individual cases of health social movements; we consider them as a collective group that when taken together have been an important force for social change. Scholars writing about individual social movements dealing with health have covered areas such as occupational safety and health (Rosner and Markowitz 1987), the women's health movement (Morgen 2002), AIDS activism (Epstein 1996) and environmental justice organizing (Bullard 1994). Other scholars, who focus more generally on changes in the health care system, point to the significance of these movements in medical history (Porter 1997) and health policy (Light 2000). Despite this significant body of research, scholars have not examined the forces that gave rise to the wide array of health social movements, nor carried out comparative analysis of these movements' different strategic, tactical and political approaches. Generally, scholars have not explored the collective development and impact the myriad health social movements have had on public health, medical research and health-care delivery. We believe there is an analytical benefit to considering the origins and impacts of HSMs collectively, and this work is part of a larger project to integrate and synthesise this material.

What explains the emergence of HSMs and their challenges to authority structures?

The scientization of decision-making
Why has this new class of health social movements emerged in the last decade? A central reason is that science and technocratic decision-making have become an increasingly dominant force in shaping social policy and regulation. Governmental and scientific demands for 'better science' in policy-making have become a significant and powerful authority used to support dominant political and socioeconomic systems. Through this 'scient-ization' (Morello-Frosch *et al.* forthcoming) of decision-making, industry exerts considerable control over debates regarding the costs, benefits and

potential risks of new technologies and industrial production by deploying scientific experts who work to ensure that battles over policy-making remain scientific, 'objective' and effectively separated from the social milieu in which they unfold (Beck 1992). The end result of this process is threefold: First, scientists are asked to answer questions that are virtually impossible to answer scientifically due to data uncertainties or the infeasibility of carrying out a study. Second, the process inappropriately frames political and moral questions (*i.e.* 'transcientific' issues) in scientific terms, thus limiting public participation in decision-making and ensuring that it becomes the purview of 'experts' (Weinberg 1972). Third, the scientisation of decision-making delegitimises the importance of those questions that may not be conducive to scientific analysis. All of these processes can exclude the public from important policy debates and diminish public capacity to participate in the production of scientific knowledge itself.

The continuing advance of societal rationalisation raises the role of objective scientific expertise above that of public knowledge for most social issues. Ironically, however, the quest for better science to inform good decision-making is often a veiled attempt to hide the politicisation of the policy process (Weiss 2004). This has been recently demonstrated in the United States by the persistent opposition of the Bush Administration to the widening scientific consensus on the question of global climate change and its attendant ecological and human health impacts (Gelbspan 1997). The Bush Administration has extended such antiscientific actions to a wide range of issues that go against consensus held by scientists, and that purge responsible scientists from expert panels and replace them with industry supporters: revoking major elements of the Clean Air Act's regulatory regime[1], allowing high mercury emissions from power plants, allowing lead industry representatives on Centers for Disease Control panels to stall lead regulation, firing pro-regulatory officials who seek to enforce existing policies (Union of Concerned Scientists 2004). The extent of such actions is so great that 60 Nobel Laureates signed a protest letter in February 2004.

In their efforts to counter this trend, health social movements have leveraged medical science and public health to marshal resources, conduct research, and produce their own scientific knowledge. Until recently, most health social movements have focused on expanding access to health care and improving the quality of health care. The latest emerging crop of HSMs, what we term *embodied health movements* (EHMs are discussed in greater detail below), are highly focused on the personal understanding and experience of illness, while often addressing some of the access concerns from earlier movements. EHMs have some notably different goals, strategies and targets from other health social movements. By using science to democratise knowledge production, embodied health movements can engage in effective policy advocacy and challenge aspects of the political economy, as well as transform traditional assumptions and lines of inquiry regarding disease causation and strategies for prevention. This emergence of EHMs has been catalysed by: growing public awareness about the limits of medical science to solve persistent health problems that are socially and economically mediated; the rise of bioethical issues and dilemmas of scientific knowledge production; and ultimately the collective drive to enhance democratic participation in social policy and regulation.

The rise of medical authority

The rise of medical authority is one of the most prominent features of modern society, involving laws and regulations concerning how professionals are empowered to make health decisions and to provide care, determination of and application of the knowledge base for medicine, and the power of medical authorities to deal with a variety of social problems that may not be primarily medical. Medical authority is tied into the broader trend we discussed above – the rise and solidification of scientific authority, in which science plays an increasing role in determining and evaluating social priorities. Medical authority has always involved varying alliances between health professionals, state agencies, corporate actors, scientists and citizen-activists. As in any dialectic relationship, increasing medical authority has occurred alongside increasing challenges to this authority. HSMs represent the transformation of sporadic and relatively unorganised challenges into formal and institutionalised opposition. In challenging scientific and medical authority structures, HSMs focus on the frequent medicalization of social problems, increasing scientization in which technical solutions are provided instead of social solutions, and a burgeoning corporatisation that takes many decisions out of people's hands, including what would be considered appropriate care.

Many scholars view authority structures as an aspect of state power, with actual or potential repressive authority. But in our modern scientized world, science and medicine have become increasingly powerful sources of authority that play a central role in supporting dominant political and socioeconomic systems. Concepts such as 'medical social control' (Zola 1972) and the 'medicalization of society' (Conrad 1992) have demonstrated how health belief systems and the practices of the health care system support and maintain existing class, race and gender inequalities. Further, the economic power of the health care system provides a key element of the modern political economy. As such, medical science has become a double-edged sword: HSMs often depend on its expertise and authority, while simultaneously challenging its social, cultural and economic dominance.

Their paradoxical relationship with medical science requires that HSMs manage their use of medical science in a way that avoids delegitimising their critique of its coercive and corruptive power. On the one hand, HSMs attempt to capitalise on the positive authority of medical science, and its perception as an agent of progress and benevolence. On the other hand, HSMs struggle to reveal the manner in which science and medicine are used as instruments of coercion. For example, in military medicine (Daniels 1969) and corporate medicine (Walsh 1987), health professionals ostensibly serving their patients' interests are in actuality servicing their institutions' needs, frequently going against the patients' interests. For example, corporate physicians in the asbestos industry hid from workers the information that they had mesothelioma caused by asbestos (Brodeur 1985). Growing awareness of biomedical abuses of authority have contributed to much distrust, as the public has learned of such phenomena as the Tuskegee syphilis experiment[2], the long history of radiation experiments and deliberate releases, the discriminatory testing of contraceptives on women in Puerto Rico, and the export to other countries of toxic substances banned in the US. At present, there is much attention to research fraud, conflict of interest in medical research and corporate influence in universities (Krimsky 2003).

In the face of such realisations, the highly-valued institutions of science and medicine come under sharper scrutiny, and social movements have mobilised powerful responses. Further, because these new realisations extend beyond the narrow boundaries of science and medicine, to include the political economy and dominant cultural values and institutions, health social movement challenges take on a very broad social critique. Even without the pressure of egregious violations, health movements propel wide-scale critiques. For example, the women's health movement pointed to sexism in so many ordinary realms of medicine that it was easy for women's health activism to forge a deep critique of patriarchy.

The public can more readily challenge science because it now has a multitude of ways to acquire and share scientific information for personal use and to promote policy change. People obtain extensive knowledge through increased interpersonal sharing of health concerns in self-help and support groups. Information is also obtained through major dissemination of scientific knowledge by the media (primarily print), and by wide access through the Internet to medical databases, research studies and regular news coverage of the challenges of research in the world of medical science. Nevertheless, the public has become more aware of the limitations of modern medical science to effectively address the persistent and most challenging health issues of the day; indeed, medical technology advances also go hand-in-hand with an increased risk of medical errors, microbial resistance to drug treatments, as well as iatrogenic complications that can lead to adverse health outcomes (Garrett 1994). Not surprisingly, this has led to the increased popularity of combining traditional medical treatments with alternative medicine (*e.g.* acupuncture, meditation and body work). Hence, the public's overall faith in medical science is moderated by the use of other avenues to disease treatment and health.

Public health research constantly reminds us that advances in modern medicine have not by themselves made the largest difference in improving the health status of diverse populations (McKeown 1976). Biomedical research, emphasising how individual risk factors predict diseases, receives the lion's share of regulatory attention, despite a significant body of research demonstrating that the health status of populations is largely determined by structural features such as race, class, income distribution, geography and other environmental factors (Krieger *et al.* 1993, Berkman and Kawachi 2000). This is exemplified by the increased prevalence of chronic diseases that are now impacting on new population groups (*e.g.* diabetes and obesity in children) and the resurgence of infectious diseases that the public and medical authorities had previously assumed had been eradicated or at least brought under control.

Finally, debates on ethical questions involving medical science have captured public attention. The advent of genetic testing for a variety of diseases has raised valid concern about the use of that information by employers to discriminate in the workplace and justify the exclusion of certain workers from insurance coverage (Shulte and Sweeny 1995, Shulte *et al.* 1997). Ethical concerns have been further fuelled by revelations of conflict of interest in the support of research by pharmaceutical firms, and the increasing power of private corporations to direct university research (Krimsky 2003). Public confidence in the integrity of scientific research has been challenged by revelations of corporations and federal agencies that violate the peer-review process or suppress the dissemination of research results that conflict with corporate economic interests (Ong and Glantz 2001, Rosenstock and Lee 2002, Greer and Steinzor 2002).

In addition, a spate of recent, highly publicised adverse events in human biomedical research has generated concerns about the ethical implications of using human subjects as research volunteers and has implicated the institutional culture at several prestigious research institutions for failing to protect study participants adequately. The 1999 death of an 18-year-old patient in a gene therapy trial at the University of Pennsylvania and the 2001 death of a healthy 24-year-old volunteer in an asthma study at Johns Hopkins University are the two cases that have received the greatest level of attention in the United States (Steinbrook 2002). In the Hopkins case, one of the criticisms levelled at the investigator and the university charged that because the volunteer was an employee in the laboratory conducting the experiment, she may have been subtly and inappropriately pressured by her employer or by her colleagues to participate in the experiment (Boston Globe 2001). These ethical concerns highlight how easily the thin veil of objectivity in medical research can be breached, despite the cardinal claim that science is essentially an objective endeavour. For the public, these problems highlight the polemical intersection of science, society and institutional culture, which ultimately paves the way for a critique of the dominant political economy and its adverse effect on the public's health.

HSMs: connecting health to socioeconomic, political and institutional concerns

Because health concerns are so pervasive throughout society, people are more likely to focus many grievances through a lens of health. For example, during an economic recession and periods of high unemployment, it is understandable that people will make demands for broader and better health insurance and for expansion of coverage to include the uninsured. Similarly, in an industrial society where environmental degradation is increasingly visible and in which the government has begun to roll back decades of environmental regulation and protection, it becomes clearer for the public to connect health with socioeconomic, political and institutional concerns and begin pushing for increased regulation of industrial production and enhanced community participation in the formation of environmental policy.

Some of this struggle for democratisation is due to social trends that provide a medium for the growth of health social movements; some of it is due to the achievements of health social movements themselves. The key is that increasing numbers of people presently believe they have the right and the authority to influence health policy, including access issues, quality of care, clinical interaction and federal funding of research. While some of that pressure occurs at the individual level, the most effective forms originate from the collective efforts of health social movements.

What conceptual tools can be applied to the study of HSMs?

When we began our exploration of HSMs a few years ago, we developed a preliminary typology that represents ideal types of HSMs, even though we understand that the goals and activities of some movements may fit into more than one of these categories. The model (Brown *et al.* 2004) aims to begin the process of analytically exploring a wide range of movements that deal with health rather than providing a rigid set of categories.

Health access movements seek equitable access to health care and improved provision of health care services. These include movements such as those seeking national health care reform, increased ability to pick specialists and extension of health insurance to uninsured people.

Embodied health movements address disease, disability or illness experience by challenging science on aetiology, diagnosis, treatment and prevention. Embodied health movements include 'contested illnesses' that are either unexplained by current medical knowledge or have environmental explanations that are often disputed. As a result, these groups organise to achieve medical recognition, treatment and/or research. Additionally, some established embodied health movements might include constituents who are not ill, but who perceive themselves as vulnerable to the disease; many breast cancer activists fit this characterisation, in joining other women who do have the disease. In addition to the breast cancer movement, this EHM category includes the AIDS movement, and the tobacco control movement.

Constituency-based health movements address health inequality and health inequity based on race, ethnicity, gender, class and/or sexuality differences.

These groups address disproportionate outcomes and oversight by the scientific community and/or weak science. They include the women's health movement, gay and lesbian health movement and environmental justice movement.

The categories of our typology are ideal types. There is often overlap with other categories. For example, the women's health movement can be seen as a constituency-based movement, but at the same time it contains elements of both access movements (*e.g.* in seeking more services for women) and embodied movements (*e.g.* in challenging assumptions about psychiatric diagnoses for premenstrual symptoms). We view this typology as simply one route into studying a new area, and we believe there are other possible typologies that can provide the same push. Indeed, one of the chapters in this volume, by Judith Allsop, Kathryn Jones and Rob Baggott, proposes a useful alternative model with the following types of HSMs: 'condition-based groups' that focus on specific conditions; 'population-based groups' concerned with all patients, carers or a specific population sub-group, such as children or ethnic minorities across a range of conditions; and 'formal alliance organisations' made up of other autonomous groups but linked by a shared interest such as genetics or long-term illness. As we work with such typologies, we are able to see what social factors are able to come into play and how well they can explain the development and outcomes of HSMs.

In focusing on the development of HSMs, the typology points to important questions about the similarities and differences in the ways the different types of HSMs develop. Our work on embodied health movements borrows concepts from social movements and science and technology studies scholars to elaborate on the mechanisms that shape the development of EHMs. For example, many health social movements have achieved the political victories described above by forging strategic connections between health and other social sectors (such as the environment). These connections enable them to overturn ineffective policies and push for more stringent regulation of industrial production that moves from a pollution control to a pollution prevention framework (Morello-Frosch 2002). Such strategic linkages can be understood in terms of the concept of 'social movement spillover' (Meyer and Whittier 1994), which points to two ways a movement can influence subsequent movements: 'by altering the political and cultural conditions it confronts in the external environment, and by changing the individuals, groups, and norms within the movement itself' (Meyer and Whittier 1994: 279).

The environmental breast cancer movement illustrates such a process. Spillover from the women's health movement, AIDS activism, and the toxic waste and environmental movements was vital to the development of a politicised collective illness identity of women with breast cancer that has enhanced their legitimacy in the eyes of policy-makers, scientists and their own emerging constituency. Many early breast cancer activists drew from their experience in the women's movement to ask whether their disease (including how it was recognised and treated) was yet another symptom of the adverse health effects of gender inequality. Likewise, many women learned key lessons from the AIDS movement, in which activists demanded that drug companies expanded their clinical trials, increased 'compassionate access' to promising experimental protocols, and pushed for more government funding of AIDS research. This crucial lesson spilled over into the breast cancer movement, which won significant increases in funding for research, representation of activists on federal and state-level research review panels, as well as the power to influence priority-setting for future scientific initiatives.

The social movement spillover that benefits the development of EHMs points to another of their characteristics. In challenging the authority of science and medicine by working both inside and outside the boundaries of biomedicine, EHMs can be seen as 'boundary movements' (a concept derived from Star and Greisemer's [1989] concept of 'boundary objects' and Gieryn's [1983] notion of 'boundary work'). In the scientized world of health care, EHMs learn to transcend traditional boundaries of social movements. They can move fluidly between lay and expert identities; for instance, raising money to fund their own research when the biomedical science research agenda does not make their cause a priority. Similarly, EHMs often rely on sympathetic scientists who, by collaborating with activists, begin to blur the boundary between actors inside and outside the scientific system. We have employed the concepts of social movement spillover and boundary movements in our analysis of embodied health movements. The typology of health social movements we introduced above begs the question of whether these conceptual tools for explaining the development and tactics of embodied health movements can be applied to the other types of HSMs in the typology.

A similar comparison across the types of HSMs, but in terms of the outcomes, would also be useful. There seem to be at least three main ways in which HSMs affect society. First, they produce changes in the health care and public health systems, both in terms of health care delivery, social policy and regulation. Second, they produce changes in medical science, through the promotion of innovative hypotheses, new methodological approaches to research and changes in funding priorities. Third, health social movements produce changes in civil society by pushing to democratise those institutions that shape medical research and policy-making (for examples of these three categories of HSMs, see Brown *et al.* 2004). Whether certain types of HSMs tend to be more or less successful in achieving one type of outcome but not others is worth further consideration.

Key issues in health social movements addressed by this volume

Rather than use the typology to categorise and introduce the contributions to this volume, we point to further questions that might be answered through the research reported here.

Where do HSMs fit within the broader cultural trend of public involvement in science? In the first chapter, David Hess points out that HSMs, as well as the professions of complementary and alternative medicine, commonly challenge the authority of medical knowledge. Hess defines the medical profession's dismissal of such challenges as 'paternalistic progressivism'. Paternalistic progressivism, he argues, has a counterpart in the claims by HSMs, and the public more broadly, that medicine is corrupted by materialistic philosophy and profitability concerns, specifically those of the pharmaceutical industry (what Hess calls 'medical devolution'). These duelling forces are resolved in what Hess calls the 'public shaping of science', 'in which there is both greater agency of social movement/lay advocacy organisations and greater recognition of the legitimacy of that agency'. Understanding the place of HSMs within the movement toward the public shaping of science, Hess argues, requires a theoretical synthesis of medical sociology and the sociology of science.

Melinda Goldner also addresses the challenges the complementary and alternative medicine movement make to the authority of medical knowledge. Unlike Hess, her focus is on the way that physicians and hospitals respond to these challenges. Like Hess, she attempts a theoretical integration of two different perspectives. In drawing on social movement and institutional theories, Goldner emphasises how health social movements can gain access to formal organisations whose boundaries are often more permeable than believed. Similarly, organisations have many ways of responding to social movement challenges. Just as Hess describes a malleable contemporary context for the negotiation of meaning in biomedical practice, Goldner describes how the outcomes of HSM activism constantly evolve depending on the negotiation between the challengers and the organisational actors.

Is there an organized 'health social movement'? In the next chapter, Judith Allsop, Kathryn Jones and Rob Baggott point us to a significant task: surveying the landscape of HSMs in order to trace the historical trend of when groups were formed, how significant they are for the whole society, and whether they coalesce into a broader 'health consumer movement'. This brings up the important distinction between social movements and social movement organisations, and leads us to think seriously about what it takes finally to determine that a larger movement exists. Allsop *et al.*'s chapter points to the emergence of a health consumer movement that crosses the lines of many different diseases and conditions. This health consumer movement is reflected in the networks and sharing of resources that exist among individual health consumer organisations.

Ganchoff's analysis of stem cell activism, which similarly points to interests held in common across a diverse set of social actors concerned with a number of different diseases and uses of stem cell research, suggests that we may need to conceive of HSMs much more broadly. Ganchoff draws on social movement theory and science and technology studies to develop the concept of a field of biotechnology. His development of this concept is significant in terms of its ability to focus analytical attention 'on a field of relationships and conflicts', which 'deepens understandings of how "biomedicalization" is operating and transforming both biomedicine and the subjects that live and move within and across its uneven and stratified terrains'. Ganchoff's conceptualisation of a field of biotechnology points to the movement actors one would expect – disease groups who stand to benefit from potential breakthroughs in stem-cell research – while also allowing him to see economic and government interests as central actors in the movement. In the end, Ganchoff's analysis also asks us to think anew about the ways in which social, political and scientific actors participate in the construction of biomedical knowledge.

In the next chapter we once again see how health social movements often result in unexpected relationships. Carole Joffe, Tracy Weitz and Clare Stacey meticulously detail the on-again-off-again relationship between abortion activists and physicians. Most recently, the vocal anti-abortion movement in the United States has created an even tighter bond between these 'uneasy allies'. Joffe *et al.* observe two tensions: one between activist doctors and a profession that may perceive them as 'fanatics', and another between committed, radical feminist activists and an increasingly professional movement. The role these tensions play in shaping the collaborations and strategies of the diverse actors in the abortion rights movement, they note, need to be studied further in related movements such as the medical marijuana and physician-assisted suicide movements.

How do full-fledged social movement organisations emerge from a hodgepodge of interest or support groups? To this point, the topics of the chapters in the volume represent fairly obvious instances of social movements. The next chapter deals with two obstacles to the further development of a health social movement. From her observations of the Alzheimer's Association in the United States, Renée Beard concludes that 'Despite the fact that encouraging more people with [Alzheimer's Disease] to speak publicly can benefit the Association's efforts, the incorporation of personal spokespersons for the AD movement suffers the same biomedical and caregiver biases as does so much of Alzheimer's research'. According to Beard, the Association's caregiver-focus and its commitment to working within the institution of biomedical research have kept it from more politicised activities. Beard's research points to important considerations for investigating other disease-based movements where the disease's pathology or the demographics of the population prevent those directly affected by the disease from representing the voice of the movement.

How do HSMs use cultural resources to achieve their goals? In contrast, Emily Kolker examines one of the most respected and successful health social movements, the breast cancer movement. But she asks a very interesting question of this movement, that can be extended to other health social movements: How do health social movements strategically use cultural resources to engage in funding activism? Her analysis points to the significance of the cultural meanings attached to disease sufferers. After all, prostate cancer activists will never be able to use the 'gender equity' or 'family erosion' claims employed by breast cancer activists as they attempted to mobilise funding for further research into breast cancer. As important, Kolker's research provides a useful contrast to the view that much health activism is about science. Though science will always be central to many HSMs' efforts, all movements take place within a broader culture where the symbolic meanings attached to diseases and people hold great significance for marshalling scientific knowledge.

The volume concludes with Maren Klawiter's fascinating exploration of one woman's breast cancer history. Klawiter meticulously illustrates how the breast cancer movement has transformed the 'regime of breast cancer' so that 'collective identities, emotional vocabularies, popular images, public policies, institutionalised practices, social scripts and authoritative discourses' give women with breast cancer today a fundamentally changed experience from 20–30 years ago. Klawiter's work is significant in terms of sociological accounts of breast cancer in that where most previous work has emphasised the movement's politicisation of breast cancer, Klawiter actually demonstrates how this politicisation alters the very experience of breast cancer for one woman. Equally important, this work represents an important advance in the study of HSMs through its focus on the implications of macro-level social movement activism on the micro-level illness experience. Future researchers should take note of Klawiter's use of transformation-of-illness experience as a measure of social movement success.

Taken together, these chapters begin to build a coherent body of evidence that HSMs are a legitimate social phenomenon while offering theoretical insight into the types of conceptual developments necessary for further analysis. The diversity of theoretical approaches must partly explain the great range of methods. At one extreme, Allsop and colleagues search for all known examples of health activism, and then use survey methods to gather information on the groups they located. At the other, Klawiter employs the illness narrative of one woman to explore the way in which the experience of breast cancer changed over time as a result of changes in the regime of breast cancer, involving changes in medicine, changes in the public visibility and mainstream awareness of breast cancer, the emergence of the breast cancer movement, and a specifically feminist politics of breast cancer. In the middle, Joffe and colleagues use archival materials, interviews and historical analysis to trace physicians' involvement in abortion rights. Similar to Beard and Goldner, Ganchoff uses interviews with activists from four social movements, websites and written material. Kolker employs content analysis of Congressional testimony, media and other texts. Finally, Hess sticks primarily to the theoretical realm. Theoretically and methodologically, the research in this volume speaks clearly to the need for integrative, and even interdisciplinary, approaches to the study of multi-layered and complex health social movements.

Conclusion

Studying health social movements offers insight into an innovative and powerful form of political action aimed at transforming the health care system, modifying people's experience of illness and addressing broader social determinants of health and disease of diverse communities. Health social movements challenge state, institutional and cultural authorities in order to enhance public participation in social policy and regulation, and to democratise the production and dissemination of scientific knowledge in medical science and public health research. In order to achieve their goals, HSMs deploy an array of strategies and are nimble in the way they shift arenas of struggle. The inter-sectoral nature of HSMs strengthens their capacity to impact on scientific and policy realms as they forge strategic alliances with movements targeting other sectors, such as the environmental movement. Finally, HSMs utilise a broad range of tactics: they engage in the legal realm, shape public health research, employ cultural resources such as popular gender norms, promote new approaches to medical science, employ creative media tactics to highlight the need for structural social change and true disease prevention and engage within the policy arena to enhance public power to monitor and regulate industrial production.

HSM activism in scientific knowledge production may also introduce potential contradictions. Although engaging in scientific endeavours is important, this process can also sap energy and staff time that might otherwise be directed toward political and community organising. Engaging in scientific activities may cause dissension among movement groups, especially if those working on collaborations with academic researchers begin to attain far more resources and institutional access than other groups. Thus, it is important to keep in mind that as activists begin to take science into their own hands, they must grapple directly with some of the same polemical issues and contradictions that they had previously criticised. For example, some health movement groups have major disagreements over whether to take corporate funding to support their work. This issue has been particularly controversial for the environmental breast cancer movement, where groups have debated whether to accept funding from major pharmaceutical firms. Some activists have argued that accepting such corporate funding can create a real or perceived conflict of interest and undermine the credibility of an organisation reliably to analyse and disseminate scientific information, especially data regarding clinical trials for new drug protocols. Other groups must address ethical quandaries, such as Native American groups that work with scientists to analyse the presence of persistent contaminants in human breast milk. In carrying out this research, activists have sought to develop informed consent procedures that address the needs of the community and not just individual community members, and they must negotiate appropriate ways to report individual and collective study results to the community (Schell and Tarbell 1998).

Despite these challenges, HSMs have successfully leveraged their embodied experience of illness and forged a new path for how social movements can effectively engage in scientific knowledge production. Thus, HSMs serve as a critical counter-authority aimed at democratising and reshaping social policy and regulation in a way that transforms the socioeconomic and political conditions that underlie distributions of health and disease among populations.

Acknowledgments

This book stems from research supported by grants to Phil Brown from the Robert Wood Johnson Foundation's Investigator Awards in Health Policy Research Program (Grant #036273) and the National Science Foundation Program in Social Dimensions of Engineering, Science, and Technology (Grant #SES-9975518).

Jon Gabe was very helpful. From the selection of chapters to recruit from the preliminary abstracts, through the review and editing process, his input was thoughtful and creative. We thank the reviewers who gave us insightful analyses of the submissions, and provided detailed recommendations for authors. The contributors were very receptive to multiple rounds of revision and editing. Our collaborators in our Contested Illnesses research group have helped shape our interest in health social movements, and have engaged in countless conversations about these issues; we are grateful to the present members (Rebecca Gasior Altman, Sabrina McCormick, Brian Mayer, Rachel Morello-Frosch and Laura Senier) and former members (Meadow Linder, Theo Luebke, Joshua Mandelbaum and Pamela Webster).

Notes

1   The Clean Air Act, enacted into law in 1970, is one of the most central components of environmental protection in the United States. Its mandate for revision of standards every five years, based on new scientific data, has led to increasing regulation of air pollution, but the Bush Administration has sought to combat that process.
2   The Tuskegee Syphilis Experiment ran for 40 years, until 1972, and is the most infamous case of unethical research in the United States. Black men were left untreated for their syphilis so that researchers could observe their pathology. The outcry over this experiment led to major developments in informed consent and other research protections.

References

Beck, U. (1992) From industrial society to the risk society: questions of survival, social structure and ecological enlightenment, *Theory, Culture and Society*, 9, 97–123.
Berkman, L. and Kawachi, I. (2000) (eds) *Social Epidemiology*. Oxford: Oxford University Press.
Boston Globe (2001) Laxity in the labs. 2 September, A6.

Brodeur, P. (1985) *Outrageous Misconduct: the Asbestos Industry on Trial*. New York: Pantheon.

Brown, P., Zavestoski, S., McCormick, S., Mayer, B., Morello-Frosch, R. and Gasior, R. (2004) Embodied health movements: uncharted territory in social movement research. *Sociology of Health and Illness*, 26, 1–31.

Bullard, R. (ed.) (1994) *Confronting Environmental Racism: Voices from the Grassroots*. Boston: South End Press.

Conrad, P. (1992) Medicalization and social control, *Annual Review of Sociology*, 18, 209–32.

Daniels, A.K. (1969) The captive professional: bureaucratic limitations in the practice of military psychiatry, *Journal of Health and Social Behavior*, 10, 255–64.

Epstein, S. (1996) *Impure Science: AIDS, Activism, and the Politics of Knowledge*. Berkeley: University of California Press.

Garrett, L. (1994) *The Coming Plague: Newly Emerging Diseases in a World Out of Balance*. New York: Farrar, Straus and Giroux.

Gelbspan, R. (1997) *The Heat Is On: the Climate Crisis, the Cover-Up, the Prescription*. Cambridge, MA: Perseus.

Gieryn, T. (1983) Boundary-work and the demarcation of science from non-science, *American Sociological Review*, 48, 781–95.

Greer, L. and Steinzor, R. (2002) Bad science. *The Environmental Forum*, January/February, 28–43.

Krieger, N., Rowley, D.L., Herman, A.A., Avery, B. and Phillips, M.T. (1993) Racism, sexism, and social class: implications for studies of health, disease, and well-being, *American Journal of Preventive Medicine*, 9, 6, 82–122.

Krimsky, S. (2003) *Science in the Private Interest: Has the Lure of Profits Corrupted Biomedical Research?* Lanham, MD: Rowman and Littlefield.

Light, D. (2000) The medical profession and organizational change: from professional dominance to countervailing power. In Bird, C., Conrad, P. and Fremont, A. (eds) *Handbook of Medical Sociology*. Upper Saddle River N.J.: Prentice Hall.

McKeown, T. (1976) *The Modern Rise of Population*. New York: Academic Press.

Meyer, D.S. and Whittier, N. (1994) Social movement spillover, *Social Problems*, 41, 277–98.

Morgen, S. (2002) *Into our Own Hands: the Women's Health Movement in the United States, 1969–1990*. New Brunswick, NJ: Rutgers University Press.

Morello-Frosch, R. (2002) The political economy of environmental discrimination, *Environment and Planning C, Government and Policy*, 20, 477–96.

Morello-Frosch, R., Zavestoski, S., Brown, P., Gasior Altman, McCormick, S. and Mayer, B. (forthcoming) Social movements in health: responses to and shapers of a changed medical world. In Moore, K. and Frickel, S. (eds) *The New Political Sociology of Science: Institutions, Networks, and Power*. Madison, WI: University of Wisconsin Press.

Ong, E.K. and Glantz, S. (2001) Constructing sound science and good epidemiology: tobacco, lawyers, and public relations firms, *American Journal of Public Health*, 91, 1749–57.

Porter, R. (1997) *The Greatest Benefit to Mankind: A Medical History of Humanity*. New York: W.W. Norton.

Rosenstock, L. and Lee, L.J. (2002) Attacks on science: the risks to evidence-based policy, *American Journal of Public Health*, 92, 14–18.

Rosner, D. and Markowitz, G. (1987) *Dying for Work: Workers' Safety and Health in Twentieth-Century America*. Indianapolis: Indiana University Press.

Schell, L. and Tarbell, A. (1998) A partnership study of PCBs and the health of mohawk youth: lessons from our past and guidelines for our future, *Environmental Health Perspectives*, 106 (Supplement 3), 833–40.

Schulte, P.A. and Sweeney, M.H. (1995) Ethical considerations, confidentiality issues, rights of human subjects, and uses of monitoring data in research and regulation, *Environmental Health Perspectives*, 103 (Supplement 3), 69–74.

Schulte, P.A., Hunter, D. and Rothman, N. (1997) Ethical and social issues in the use of biomarkers in epidemiological research, in application of biomarkers in cancer epidemiology. *International Agency for Research on Cancer*, Lyon, France, 313–18.

Seale, C. (2003) Health and media: an overview, *Sociology of Health and Illness*, 25, 6, 513–31.

Star, S.L. and Greisemer, K. (1989) Institutional ecology, 'translations,' and boundary objects: amateurs and professionals in Berkeley's Museum of Vertebrate Zoology, 1907–39, *Social Studies of Science*, 19, 387–420.

Steinbrook, R. (2002) Protecting research subjects – the crisis at Johns Hopkins. *New England Journal of Medicine*, 346, 716–20.

Union of Concerned Scientists (2004) *Scientific Integrity in Policymaking: an Investigation into the Bush Administration's Misuse of Science*. Cambridge, MA: Union of Concerned Scientists.

Walsh, D.C. (1987) *Corporate Physicians: between Medicine and Management*. New Haven: Yale University Press.

Weinberg, A. (1972) Science and transcience, *Minerva*, 10, 2, 209–22.

Weiss, R. (2004) Peer review plan draws criticism under Bush proposal, OMB would evaluate science before new rules take effect, *Washington Post*, 15 January, 2004, A19.

Zola, I.K. (1972) Medicine as an instrument of social control, *Sociological Review*, 20, 487–504.

Chapter 2

Medical modernisation, scientific research fields and the epistemic politics of health social movements
David J. Hess

Introduction

How has the emergence of health social movements (HSMs) altered the relationships among the medical research community and the public? The question is somewhat foreign in the context of North American social movement (SM) theories, which tend to focus on movement dynamics, but it does have some parallels with European studies of new SMs (*e.g.* Habermas 1987, Touraine 1992, cf. Pichardo 1997) and their role in reflexive modernisation (Beck 1992, 1996). This chapter develops the hypothesis that modern scientific medicine is undergoing increasing challenges to its epistemic authority, in part due to the rise of health SMs and in part due to the growth of 'complementary and alternative medicine' (CAM), and that those challenges have brought about institutional and epistemic changes that are described here as 'medical modernisation'. The argument goes beyond the study of lay expertise (Prior 2003) to investigate how HSMs affect medical research communities.

The patterns described for such epistemic challenges are drawn primarily from the author's decade of research on science and the CAM cancer therapy movement in the US (*e.g.* Hess 1997, 1999). The field of CAM is a complex amalgam of reformers within the medical profession and associated research communities, industries and government bodies, as well as alternative healthcare professions, lay healers and patient-advocacy organisations. In the US since the 1970s some CAM organisations have coalesced into a CAM cancer therapy movement that has raised significant challenges to the epistemic authority of medical expertise (Hess 2003, Markle and Peterson 1980). Similar patterns of challenge to medical expertise can be found in other disease-based HSMs (*e.g.* Brown *et al.* 2001, 2002, Clarke 1998, Epstein 1996, Kroll-Smith and Floyd 1997). Their previous research is built upon here to develop further the emergent synthesis between medical sociology and the sociology of science. Such a synthesis is needed to understand the implications that the epistemic challenges of HSMs pose to the medical profession and medical research communities.

Conceptual background

Modernity is understood here not as a specific series of events (*e.g.* the Scientific Revolution, the Enlightenment, the Industrial Revolution) but, instead, as the ongoing development of a system of institutions that includes representative democracy, legal universalism, private markets, religious and intellectual pluralism, and social mobility. The relationship between medicine and modernity can be traced back to the rise of empiricism and experimentalism in the 17th century, but it is more often associated with the rise of institutionalised biomedical research in the late 19th century, its adoption by a medical profession, and the development of state support for the hegemony of biomedical research and the medical profession over competing medical systems (Starr 1982). In the late 20th century, a second issue emerged in the historical sociology of medicine: the decline of professional dominance and the rise of countervailing powers (Light 2000).

Although the term 'medical modernisation' could be used to refer to a variety of historical changes in medicine, the focus here is on its epistemic dimension. Specifically, the hypothesis is that since the 1960s the medical profession and affiliated research communities have undergone institutional and epistemic changes in response to knowledge challenges mounted by CAM and HSMs. Not all advocates of CAM and HSMs pose such challenges. Some CAM advocates do not generate empirical research or participate in the basic assumptions of modern science. Likewise, some HSMs, such as movements around health-care equity, do not touch the third rail of the legitimacy of therapeutic and knowledge consensus in medicine. As Brown and colleagues (2002) note, scientific knowledge plays a greater role in the HSMs that are based on disease. In disease-based social movements, patients experience a disjuncture between their 'illness' (Kleinman 1981) and the diagnostic and therapeutic world of 'disease', or the official systems of aetiology and treatment.

Patients have long experienced scepticism toward their doctors, but they have tended to live with medical expertise due to their sense of dependence, a pattern that is found in other confrontations between lay and expert knowledge (Wynne 1996). With the rise of disease-oriented HSMs and counter-expertise, there is a historical change in the epistemic status of the patient. This can be understood as the 'death of the patient' in the original, etymological sense of the term 'patient' as someone who endures. The title of the book by one breast cancer patient-advocate, *Patient No More* (Batt 1994), aptly signals the change from patient to knowledge-challenging activist. The cogito of patient-based knowledge – 'I am not getting better; therefore, I doubt' – is very old, but in the crucible of patient advocacy organisations, CAM professions and counter-experts within medical research communities, the cogito becomes transmuted into an epistemic challenge. The type of expertise goes beyond the experiential knowledge of individual patients about their bodies and illness experience to a coalition or hybridisation of experiential knowledge, lay expertise and counter-expertise (Fischer 2000, Jamison 2001).

It is beyond the scope of this chapter to develop an explanation of why such changes have occurred. Clearly, the changes need to be explained with reference to broader societal processes, such as reflexive modernisation, but a few suggestions specific to the medical field can be made here. First, the successes of medicine (*e.g.* the epidemiological transition of mortality in developed countries toward chronic, non-infectious diseases; the ageing of the population; the medicalization of previously non-medical dimensions of life; and the discovery of new diseases and aetiological agents) have created an ongoing gap between expectations and delivery that undermines modernist rhetoric about an impending era in which the progress of medicine will eradicate disease. Second, the accumulation of reports of iatrogenic disease, hospital errors, and capture of medical science by profit motives has led to increased scepticism and civil society mobilisation, which in turn have been facilitated by the rise of the Internet and other forms of mass communication. Third, the medical profession and research communities themselves have grown and differentiated, creating the conditions for more controversy, while at the same time some of the CAM professions, such as chiropractors and naturopathic physicians in the US, have developed scientific research programmes and in other ways undergone professionalization (Baer 2001).

As challenges increase to the epistemic authority of the medical profession and healthcare research community, a response is required. It is helpful to compare the situation with the environmental sociology literature on responses to challenges to industrial production wrought by emergent environmental knowledge. One type of response is denial, suppression, and retrenchment around traditional brown industries of the 'treadmill of production' (Schnaiberg and Gould 1994). At the opposite extreme is a community-oriented withdrawal from global systems, in which activists attempt to create alternative, locally-oriented institutions such as home power and community-supported agriculture. In between is a complex middle terrain of 'ecological modernisation', in which the private sector undergoes a partial greening of production that is monitored and spurred by the state and civil society (Hajer 1996, Mol and Spaargaren 2000).

In a similar way, the challenge of alternative knowledge claims about disease has created different types of response. The first, termed here 'paternalistic progressivism', is found most frequently in the medical research elite and in the anti-CAM 'quackbusters', who emphasise the purity of scientific medical knowledge and the lack of value in epistemic challenges from CAM and HSMs (*e.g.* Herbert 1994). They reinforce the boundary work that sets up the cultural equivalence that science is to biomedical knowledge as non-science is to the knowledge of patients and CAM providers. At the other extreme is the rejection of conventional medicine, usually built around its failures in the treatment of chronic diseases such as cancer, and found in the radical alternative wings of CAM movements. This approach, termed here 'medical devolution', views scientific medicine as corrupted by materialistic philosophy and financial interests, specifically those of the pharmaceutical industry, and in need of fundamental change in its epistemic assumptions (*e.g.* Culbert 1994).

The term 'medical modernisation' is used here, in parallel with ecological modernisation, to signal an emergent third type of response. The response is emerging in part because of the legitimation crisis that occurs with the development of counter-expertise, but also because of the effects that the epistemic challenges of HSMs and CAM professionals have on funding agendas and patients' spending preferences. Known as 'integrative' medicine in the clinical setting, the term 'medical modernisation' includes the knowledge and research dimension of the challenge of integrating or rebuffing epistemic challenges. Evidence-based medicine and science become the points of reference in resolving disputes over how medicine is to be integrated and which therapies are to be accepted or rejected. At the same time, methodologies and funding priorities become more closely inspected for bias, and hence scientific research becomes both more important and more subject to political dispute. As with ecological modernisation for green technologies, the more complementary therapies are selected to be used in an adjuvant mode, but the fundamental therapeutic repertoire of medicine is in many cases largely untouched (Hess forthcoming).

The shifting field of epistemic power relations around the alternative knowledges produced in HSMs, CAM professions, and non-dominant biomedical research networks is by no means uniform. As Zavestoski et al. (2002) note, persons with Gulf War-related illnesses (Brown et al. 2001), multiple chemical sensitivity (Kroll-Smith and Floyd 1997), and other contested diseases face epistemic challenges largely around the existence of their diseases. In contrast, because AIDS or breast cancer patients start with recognition of the existence of their disease, their epistemic challenges rest more on treatment options. The CAM-oriented patients and clinicians often mount challenges around different conceptions of aetiology that feed into alternative or complementary therapies. Notwithstanding the differences, across a wide range of diseases the medical research community faces the similar problem of rebuffing, accepting or modifying alternative ways of knowing and networks of counter-expertise.

Epistemic challenges to medicine are by no means new, but as the challengers increasingly press their claims with reference to modern science, the conditions for medical modernisation emerge. As a result, the distinction between lay/alternative knowledge and scientific knowledge, upon which the epistemic authority of medicine rested, is submerged in a more complex field of competing scientific networks and research programmes. Rather than view the current form of epistemic conflicts as 'lay knowledge' in the disease-based HSMs that is either rejected or accepted by the 'expert knowledge' in the medical research communities, the argument here is that the social scientist needs a more complex model of scientific research fields that emphasises their inherent pluralism. Because the professionalised CAM systems have their own research communities, journals and domains of expertise, and because leaders of HSMs develop expertise and partnerships with non-dominant research networks both within biomedicine and in the CAM professions, an adequate theoretical framework needs to synthesise medical sociology and the sociology of scientific research fields.

The modernisation of scientific research fields

As an institution, science is also undergoing a modernisation process that has significant theoretical implications. Many of the mid-20th-century theories of science, including the work of Kuhn (1970), assumed a level of autonomy for scientific research fields that was probably inaccurate at the time but certainly is no longer credible today. Changes in the academic and private-sector research-and-development enterprises have increasingly whittled away at the autonomy of research fields. Increasingly, researchers are offered incentives to enhance their level of external funding and to develop research products that can be patented and licenced (Kleinman 2003). Terms such as 'academic capitalism' (Slaughter and Leslie 1997) and 'mode-2 knowledge production' (Gibbons *et al.* 1994) have emerged in the literature to describe the transformation. Tie-ins to industry provide opportunities for new sources of funding when state funding agency and foundation budgets are flat, and private-sector sponsorship also provides greater potential for partnerships leading to technology transfer. Although it is debatable that in fields such as physics, chemistry, engineering and medicine there ever was a strong level of autonomy (Kevles 1997, Noble 1977), the autonomy model is increasingly inaccurate given the significant institutional changes that have occurred in scientific knowledge production.

By giving up the autonomy assumption, one develops a model of the social shaping of knowledge that grapples with two related problems: how research fields are shaped at a broad, macro level and which science is completed versus which science is left undone. When researchers select a 'research programme' to work on – that is, a combination of research problem area, method and conceptual framework – they are simultaneously positioning themselves socially as part of various research networks that operate along those three dimensions. For example, if one takes cancer treatment as a broad problem area, the researchers and research programmes that work in this problem area also connect outward along the other two dimensions to various conceptual frameworks anchored in subdisciplines, as well as to methods that may cross disciplines and subdisciplines. The plurality of actors' positions makes it possible for one research culture to challenge another, so that a claim to scientific expertise can unravel, particularly when internal challengers have allies in external institutions or SMs.

Research fields are comprised of research networks that are related to each other by patterns of conflict and co-operation that shift over time, rather than being dominated by a single paradigm that undergoes occasional shifts (Fuller 2000). Although in the short run some research fields may achieve a Kuhnian level of consensus agreement on the important research problems, methods and concepts, such conditions would lead rapidly to stagnation due to the problem of diminishing returns of research to a method applied to the same problem area (Rescher 1978). Rather, it is more typical for a research field to be characterised by competing knowledge claims rooted in contrasting methods and conceptual frameworks. Yet, all is not anarchy or a level playing field of pluralistic research networks; hence, the paradigm concept does flag a condition that is frequently seen. It is often the case that research fields have one or more dominant networks that control the lion's share of resources in the field. In medicine the pattern has been described as the 'dominant epidemiological paradigm' (Brown *et al.* 2001, Zavestoski *et al.* 2002). The terms dominant 'networks' or 'research programmes' are preferred here to emphasise the pluralism and conflict in research fields. Although there are dominant and non-dominant networks in most research fields, the dominant networks are constantly undergoing colonisation efforts by new networks of researchers who are importing new methods or concepts for a problem, or who are attempting to divert resources for a method or conceptual framework to new problem areas. Controversy is therefore not a sign of the pathology of science but of its vigorous vetting process through complex linkages of co-operation and competition. In other words, controversy over what the important problems should be, what the best methods are, and how the problems should be defined are part of 'normal' science, not, as Kuhnians would argue, symptoms of the preparadigmatic phase of an immature science.

Controversies can be resolved internally by negotiation and iterative research among the competing networks, but outside actors often intervene before the closure process works itself out (Collins 2002: 246). For example, funders need to make decisions about which research programmes need funding, and thus closure may be enforced by related communities of experts who are not part of the core set of parties to a conflict, but who, in the terms presented here, may share one or more of the research cultures with the core set (problem area, methods, concepts). In the medical field, health SMs and CAM professions provide an example of an economic basis for funding opportunities that can help open and close controversies.

The expansion of therapeutic nutrition, which has had a major role in the CAM cancer therapy movement, provides a helpful example. Nutritional interventions are accepted medical knowledge for the prevention of many diseases and the treatment of a small number of recognised nutritional deficiency diseases, but they remain highly controversial when used for the treatment of some of the most common chronic diseases. In the US, HSM pressure helped spur the development of funding through the National Center for Complementary and Alternative Medicine of the National Institutes of Health, but funding also came through the CAM schools, research-oriented clinicians, the food and supplements industry, and some biochemical and nutrition science researchers who devoted part of their research portfolio to studies of therapeutic nutrition for chronic disease. The inflow of resources helped the therapeutic nutrition networks to mount an increasing and sustained challenge to the dominant research networks of patentable, drug-based research on therapies for chronic disease. Over time, the alternative knowledges accumulated and were packed down in review essays and consensus statements. The build-up of knowledge tended to overwhelm the claims of paternalistic progressives and other sceptics who rejected the idea that therapeutic nutrition can be valuable for the treatment or cure of chronic diseases such as cancer. They become increasingly isolated voices, but at the same time the more radical critics in the CAM movements, who may be anchored in the experiential knowledge of clinical practice but do not produce research, also become isolated.

The older rhetorical battles between the paternalistic progressives and medical devolutionists increasingly take on an archaic ring. In their wake a series of new research projects emerges around the integration of drugs and therapeutic nutrition, and even around new classes of entities (nutraceuticals), as the alternative knowledge claims that were once on the outside (embedded in patient advocacy organizations and CAM professional networks) now become incorporated and transformed into mainstream knowledge and practice. Thus, in contrast to the view that the alternative epistemic claims of the HSMs and CAM professions become, in a sense, hypotheses that medical research communities may either investigate or ignore, the model described here views the challenging claims as a process of integration that occurs through the growth of alternative research networks and the triggering and closure of scientific controversies.

The demise of the transmission policy

The emergence of a middle ground between expert and lay knowledge in the form of alternative research networks has contributed to the demise of a policy model that defines the ideal relationship between medical research and 'the public'. Under the policy model of transmission or diffusion, research communities produce expert knowledge that is then diffused to the public. In turn, an appreciative public sends a message to public funding agencies and private foundations to continue to fund scientific research. As public support of scientific research became more precarious during the last decades of the 20th century, the transmission policy has increasingly turned to the problem of scientific literacy in the general public. Surveys showed that the public understanding of science was very low and that the public suffered from a problem of scientific illiteracy. The remedy, under the transmission policy, is more science education and better communication of science to the public.

The transmission policy model is based on several assumptions that have increasingly been called into question. For example, it assumes that the 'public' is a relatively undifferentiated and passive mass whose major role is to provide tacit or explicit approval of funding for scientific research. Its agency is restricted to identifying broad shifts in funding contours, usually via representatives such as members of governmental oversight committees. In contrast, many qualitative studies, mostly by sociologists and anthropologists, have developed an alternative to the transmission policy that is based on an assumption of a more active public that 'reconstructs' scientific knowledge (Brown and Mikkelson 1990, Hess 1995: ch. 6, Irwin and Wynne 1996). This view also recognises a concept of the public that is more differentiated, with pockets of literacy and illiteracy that are strategically based on need to know (Hess 1999: 229). Those pockets may take the form of geographically-based local knowledge, experientially-based knowledge such as that of patients, or combinations of both, such as communities that are suffering the health effects of toxic exposure. In turn, the reconstruction or intellectual challenge to expert knowledge can lead to a more activist approach to scientific research that emphasises the 'public shaping of science' (Hess 1999: 230). There are two major forms in which the public shaping of science occurs.

In the indirect form, the public shaping of science is largely limited to contributions to the media or to engagement with the policy process and funding decisions. Usually the work involves a splitting of the social movement or advocacy groups into some people who have developed the appropriate literacy to engage the policy and funding communities; in other words, they have undergone an 'expertification' process (Epstein 1996). The nature of the expertise of the 'lay experts' is generally what I have called 'narrow-band competence' (Hess 1999: 229); the activists are competent in a narrow research programme but tend to lack the broader knowledge of a technical discipline or a research problem area that is typical of scientific researchers. As a result, they can fall off the 'knowledge cliff' fairly easily (Forsythe 2001). However, they are competent enough to engage in the policy and public opinion networks that shape funding, and, if successful, they can bring about shifts in funding priorities across or within research fields. Nevertheless, the outcomes of the shifts in funding may not be what the patients want; often the research communities recapture or rechannel the funding (Brown et al. 2001, Clarke 1998, Hess 2002).

In the direct form of the public shaping of science, activists/advocates make the transition to the status of contributors to scientific research fields by helping to develop new research programmes that are aligned with their goals but are at odds with the dominant research programmes of the research fields. In my historical and ethnographic research on the CAM cancer therapy movement, three basic types of mechanisms became evident: 'conversion', biographical transformation and network assemblage. Similar mechanisms can be found in other health social movements, such as the AIDS movement (Epstein 1996) and Gulf War Illness veterans' movement (Zavestoski et al. 2002), so these mechanisms are probably generalisable across HSMs that mount epistemic challenges.

In conversion, activists convince scientists who are working in a dominant research programme to shift to a research programme aligned with the activists' goals. In the CAM cancer therapy movement, the successful recruitment of high-power researchers from the dominant networks is relatively rare, but I observed some cases of conversion of dominant-network researchers when they were battling terminal cancer. The nature of the conversions tended to be weak, that is, toward the complementary end of the therapeutic spectrum. The pattern observed in the CAM cancer movement is similar to one observed in the environmental movement, where conversions were easily accomplished with emeritus and retired researchers who were no longer dependent on the funding pipeline and could therefore afford to take the risks associated with the politics of counter-expertise (Downey 1988). Another type of conversion that occurred in the CAM cancer therapy movement took place when accredited researchers developed alternative research programmes and therapies that resulted in suppression and their subsequent political awakening.

A second mechanism represents an extreme variation of the expertification process that permits direct involvement in scientific research: the biographical transformation of activists/advocates into researchers through additional education. Patient-activists can pass through an entire trajectory or conveyer belt of role transitions: from disatisfied patients to clients of alternative practitioners, to members and leaders of patient-advocacy organisations, to the lay researchers whom Epstein (1996) described, and finally to graduate students and healthcare professionals and researchers. In examining biographical trajectories among CAM cancer therapy activists in the US, patient-activists may stop at any point on the way, and very few actually complete the transition into the final stage. In other words, there is a funnel process in which many make the first transition, fewer the second, and even fewer go on to become accredited practitioners or researchers.

The third mechanism of the direct form of the public shaping of science, network assemblage, is more common, at least in the CAM cancer therapy movement in the US. Here, activists/advocates help weave together networks of patients, funding sources, clinicians and potential researchers, and they sometimes write review essays and books that are significant contributions to the field. Examples are the work of the Gerson Research Organization, Commonweal, the Center for Advancement in Cancer Education, the Moss Reports, and the National Foundation for Alternative Medicine. The leaders of those organisations do not have medical degrees, but they are accomplished professionals in some other field. In several cases, leaders of CAM patient advocacy organisations have graduate educations in fields such as the social sciences, and consequently they possess the tacit knowledge involved in doing scientific research. In some cases the activist/researcher becomes the lead author or co-author in a journal publication that advances the research field; the articles can be review essays or presentations of new data, such as those culled from CAM clinicians' records (*e.g.* Hildenbrand *et al.* 1996). As is common in science, publications are usually co-authored with various experts contributing to different parts of the research project.

Whether the public shaping of science occurs indirectly through the funding-policy networks or directly via the challenge to the dominant research programmes within a research field, the outcome of activist involvement in science will tend to produce controversy. If activists become aligned with non-dominant research programmes and bring to them new resources, they can invigorate the resource position of the non-dominant networks. Historically, the researchers in the dominant networks have tended to engage in a wide variety of suppression tactics aimed at activists, clinicians and researchers who have departed from the dominant research programmes. Suppression includes campaigns to subject challengers to dismissal or litigation, funding cuts to challenging research networks and media campaigns to discredit challengers (Martin 1999). Some of the veteran CAM cancer therapy activists have referred to occasional 'pincer movements' in which a variety of suppression mechanisms were brought to bear simultaneously. The worst of suppression may be reserved for the high-status insiders turned critic-challengers, such as Linus Pauling (Richards 1981) or Peter Duesberg (Epstein 1996), but it is also directed at clinicians who become too famous, and it creates a chilling effect for other would-be challengers. The suppression strategy tends to be correlated with the ideological response of paternalistic progressivism, in which there is a blanket rejection of challenging knowledge claims. In some cases HSM mobilisation and public pressure from dissident scientists have forced the release of funding for clinical trials, but in such cases the suppression strategy can extend into manipulation of experimental design to introduce biases against the CAM therapy (Moss 1996, Richards 1981). The evidence for bias and suppression feeds the radical critiques of the medical devolution side of the CAM clinicians and patient advocates.

Under conditions of medical modernisation, the older dynamic of suppression and outcries of corruption are replaced by the institutionalised incorporation of challenging epistemic claims into the formation of new research fields, and the incorporation of alternative researchers into funded research programmes with principal investigator status. Although the policy of transmission and suppression was still evident even in the first decade of the 21st century, there was increasing institutionalisation of the voices of patients and scientifically-oriented CAM advocates into the research process. What once took a SM to open up research policymaking to public debate (AIDS, breast cancer, CAM cancer therapies, etc.) is now increasingly institutionalised through the conversion of SM organisations into insider patient-advocacy organisations with their client-research networks. Obviously, the modernisation of patient advocacy also entails a degree of capture and control, and the complexities of co-optation are as great as in the environmental movement (Jamison 2001). More generally, the institutionalisation of SMs into interest groups has long been recognised as one general outcome when elites recognise the need for changes that integrate movement demands (Zald and Ash 1966). The argument here is a more specific one about a point in the historical development of the modern medical field, in which there are signs of an opening to epistemic challenges (patients' experiences, CAM systems) when cast as scientific research programmes, and a concomitant transformation of the politics of suppression into one of incorporation.

Conclusion

This chapter develops the hypothesis that epistemic challenges to medical knowledge have resulted in an institutional response that is described here as part of 'medical modernisation'. The focus has been on the relations between biomedical research communities and epistemic challenges mounted by some categories of HSMs and CAM. A more complete analysis would be needed to explore the relations between those two types of actors and the industries that develop the technologies – pharmaceutical, nutraceutical (supplements), radiation, etc. – as well as the providers of clinical care. Another problem is the comparative study of the relations among knowledge-producing communities, social movements/lay activists, product-producing communities and product-utilising communities in other health social movements and other technology- and product-oriented movements (see Hess forthcoming). A third area worthy of further study is the relative geographical scope of the hypothesis of medical modernisation. The epistemic challenges of disease-based HSMs may be relatively unique to the individualism of the US and similar political cultures, but the epistemic challenges mounted by research-oriented CAM professions are much more international. Consequently, one would expect that similar processes occur in many countries, but that they are also subject to substantial variation. Yet another topic worth further exploration is the co-optation process of both patient advocacy groups and the CAM professions, such as chiropractors and naturopathic doctors in the US. The issue would entail not only the manipulation and capture of patient advocacy organisations and some CAM professions, but also internal divisions between their accommodationist and radical wings.

The general argument presented here is that as the voices of patients, CAM professionals, and their allied networks of non-dominant researchers and providers are incorporated into the medical mainstream, the importance of science does not recede but instead grows, even as it becomes more contentious. Rather than ignore patients and suppress rogue researchers and clinicians, the modernisation process increasingly provides some funding (albeit limited), a challenge to substantiate their claims with scientific research, and a promise to integrate scientifically-vetted epistemic claims. As a result, medical sociology needs to face the challenge of continued integration with the sociology of science, specifically the social, historical and cultural studies of scientific knowledge. To do so, one needs to explore the knowledge-making coalitions that emerge among HSMs, non-dominant networks and sources of funding that can lead to consensus shifts in the research communities.

References

Baer, H. (2001) *Biomedicine and Alternative Healing Systems in America*. Madison, Wi.: University of Wisconsin Press.
Batt, S. (1994) *Patient No More*. Charlottetown, P.E.I., Canada: Gynergy Books.
Beck, U. (1992) *The Risk Society*. London and Beverly Hills, Ca.: Sage.
Beck, U. (1996) Risk society and the provident state. In Lash, Scott, Szerszynski, Bronislaw, and Wynne, Brian (eds) *Risk, Environment, and Modernity*. Thousand Oaks, Ca.: Sage.
Brown, P. and Mikkelsen, E. (1990) *No Safe Place*. Berkeley, Ca.: University of California Press.
Brown, P., Zavestoski, S. and McCormick, S. (2001) A gulf of differences: disputes over Gulf-War related illness, *Journal of Health and Social Behavior*, 42, 3, 235–57.
Brown, P., Zavestoski, S., McCormick, S. and Mayer, B. (2002) Health social movements: unchartered territory in social movement research. Paper presented at the Authority in Contention Conference of the American Sociological Association, section on Collective Behavior and Social Movements, Notre Dame.
Clarke, A. (1998) *Disciplining Reproduction*. Berkeley, Ca.: University of California Press.
Collins, H.R. (2002) The third wave of science studies: studies of expertise and experience, *Social Studies of Science*, 32, 2, 235–96.
Culbert, M. (1994) *Medical Armageddon, Volumes 1 and 2*. San Diego: C&C Communications.
Downey, G. (1988) Structure and practice in the cultural identities of scientists: negotiating nuclear wastes in New Mexico, *Anthropological Quarterly*, 61, 1, 26–38.
Epstein, S. (1996) *Impure Science*. Berkeley, Ca.: University of California Press.
Fischer, F. (2000). *Citizens, Experts, and the Environment*. Durham, N.C.: Duke University Press.
Forman, P. (1987) Behind quantum electronics: national security as a basis for physical research in the U.S., 1940–1960, *Historical Studies in the Physical Sciences*, 18, 149–229.
Forsythe, D. (2001) *Studying Those Who Study Us*. Stanford, Ca.: Stanford University Press.
Fuller, S. (2000) *Thomas Kuhn: A Philosophical History for Our Times*. Chicago: University of Chicago Press.
Gibbons, M., Limoges, C. and Nowotny, H. (1994) *The New Production of Knowledge*. London: Sage.
Habermas, J. (1987) *A Theory of Communicative Action, Volume 2: Lifeworld and System*. Boston: Beacon.
Hajer, M. (1996) Ecological modernization as cultural politics. In Lash, S., Szerszynski, B. and Wynne, B. (eds) *Risk, Environment, and Modernity*. Thousand Oaks, Ca.: Sage.

Herbert, V. (1994) Three stakes in hydrazine sulfate's heart, but questionable cancer remedies, like vampires, always rise again. *Journal of Clinical Oncology*, 12, 6, 1107–08.

Hess, D. (1995) *Science and Technology in a Multicultural World*. New York: Columbia University Press.

Hess, D. (1997) *Can Bacteria Cause Cancer?* New York: NYU Press.

Hess, D. (1999) *Evaluating Alternative Cancer Therapies*. New Brunswick, N.J.: Rutgers U. Press.

Hess, D. (2002) Stronger versus weaker integration policies, *American Journal of Public Health*, 92, 10, 1579–81.

Hess, D. (2003) CAM cancer therapies in twentieth-century North America: examining continuities and change. In Johnston, R. (ed.) *The Politics of Healing*. New York: Routledge.

Hess, D. (forthcoming) Technology-approximating and product-oriented movements: social movement studies and STS, *Science, Technology, and Human Values*.

Hildenbrand, G., Hildenbrand, L.C., Bradford, K., Rogers, D., Straus, C., and Cavin, S. (1996) The role of follow-up and retrospective data analysis in alternative cancer management: The Gerson experience, *Journal of Naturopathic Medicine*, 6, 1, 49–56.

Irwin, A. and Wynne, B. (eds) (1996) *Misunderstanding Science?* Cambridge, U.K.: Cambridge University Press.

Jamison, A. (2001) *The Making of Green Knowledge*. Cambridge: Cambridge University Press.

Kevles, D. (1997) *The Physicists*. New York: Vintage.

Kleinman, A. (1981) *Patients and Healers in the Context of Culture*. Berkeley, Ca.: University of California Press.

Kleinman, D. (2003) *Impure Cultures*. Madison, Wi.: University of Wisconsin Press.

Kroll-Smith, S. and Floyd, H. (1997) *Bodies in Protest*. New York: NYU Press.

Kuhn, T. (1970) *The Structure of Scientific Revolutions*. Chicago: University of Chicago Press.

Light, D. (2000) The medical profession and organizational change: from professional dominance to countervailing power. In Bird, C., Conrad, P. and Fremont, A. (eds) *Handbook of Medical Sociology*. Upper Saddle River, N.J.: Prentice Hall.

Markle, G., and Peterson, J. (1980) *Politics, Science, and Cancer*. Washington, D.C.: American Association for the Advancement of Sciences.

Martin, B. (1999) Suppression of dissent in science. In Freudenburg, W. and Young, T. (eds) *Research in Social Problems and Public Policy, Volume 7*. Stamford, CT: JAI Press.

Mol, A. and Spaargaren, G. (2000) Ecological modernisation theory in debate: a review. In Mol, A. and Sonnenfeld, D. (eds) *Ecological Modernization Theory Around the World*. London and Portland, Or.: Frank Cass.

Moss, R. (1996) *The Cancer Industry*. Brooklyn, N.Y.: Equinox Press.

Noble, D. (1977) *America by Design*. Oxford, U.K.: Oxford University Press.

Pichardo, N. (1997) New social movements: a critical review, *Annual Review of Sociology*, 23, 411–30.

Prior, L. (2003) Belief, knowledge, and expertise: the emergence of the lay expert in medical sociology, *Sociology of Health and Illness*, 25, 3, 41–57.

Rescher, N. (1978) *Scientific Progress*. Pittsburgh, Pa.: University of Pittsburgh Press.

Richards, E. (1981) *Vitamin C and Cancer*. New York: St. Martin's.

Schnaiberg, A. and Gould, K. (1994) *Environment and Society*. New York: St. Martin's.

Slaughter, S. and Leslie, L. (1997) *Academic Capitalism*. Baltimore: The Johns Hopkins University Press.

Starr, P. (1982) *The Social Transformation of American Medicine*. New York: Basic Books.

Touraine, A. (1992) Beyond social movements? *Theory, Culture, and Society*, 9, 1, 125–45.

Wynne, B. (1996) May the sheep safely graze? A reflexive view of the expert-lay knowledge divide. In Lash, S., Szerszynski, B. and Wynne, B. (eds) *Risk, Environment, and Modernity*. Thousand Oaks, Ca.: Sage.

Zald, M. and Ash, R. (1966) Social movement organizations: growth, decay, and change, *Social Forces*, 44, 3, 327–40.

Zavestoski, S., Brown, P., Linder, M., McCormick, S. and Mayer, B. (2002) Science, policy, activism, and war: defining the health of Gulf War veterans, *Science, Technology, and Human Values*, 27, 2, 171–205.

Chapter 3

The dynamic interplay between Western medicine and the complementary and alternative medicine movement: how activists perceive a range of responses from physicians and hospitals
Melinda Goldner

Introduction

Physicians and hospitals respond to the complementary and alternative medicine (CAM) movement in the United States in multiple ways. Thus, activists perceive each outcome differently, and engage in ongoing attempts to shape these organisational responses[1]. Until recently, activists competed with physicians by providing an alternative medical model. This 'outsider' strategy was successful since consumers were increasingly frustrated by poor results and care (*Time* 1996). Established actors took notice of a study showing that 34 per cent of adults had tried at least one form of CAM (Eisenberg *et al.* 1993), because consumer usage was much higher than expected. Consequently, the federal government began to fund research on techniques like acupuncture and massage, more physicians began to refer patients to alternative practitioners or learn these techniques, hospital administrators started to integrate these techniques, and insurance companies started to reimburse patients for their use. Even though these developments represent new opportunities for the CAM movement, some activists fear losing control over their ideas and techniques (Goldner 2001). This study uses social movement and institutional theories to examine the diverse ways that organisational actors respond to the CAM movement, and in turn, how activists perceive each response.

CAM should be conceptualised as a social movement, because of the number of people identifying as activists and the collective impact they are achieving (Goldner 1999). Most practitioners and clients interviewed define their participation as activism. Though their resistance typically entails individual acts, activists are having a larger impact since they identify with a seemingly cohesive social movement that challenges Western medicine collectively. This collective effort has led to the healthcare changes outlined here. Some activist organisations lobby on behalf of the movement. Yet the CAM movement does not have one identifiable organisation that unifies the entire movement. Rather, it is a diffuse movement comprising diverse clinics, activist organisations and individuals. Activists are united through their ideology, which allows diverse and often disconnected individuals to have shared meanings, similar experiences and, most importantly, a connection to something larger than their individual participation.

Using data from California activists and hospitals in New York and Massachusetts, I develop a model specifying the range of responses the institution of Western medicine has towards the CAM movement. I only chronicle the responses of physicians and hospitals. Past studies have told us more about how consumers are responding to CAM than practitioners. Now it is important to study how CAM is developing clinically, because this is where change is now occurring. Physicians' responses are crucial since they have greater access to consumers and more power than activists (Cant and Sharma 2000, Yoshida 2002). Since physicians are the main actors in hospitals it is important to study these organisations as a new site of CAM. These organisational actors can avoid, compromise with, acquiesce, manipulate or defy the demands of the CAM movement.

Activists attempt to direct institutionalisation[2] since CAM is not completely incorporated into Western medicine (Adams and Tovey 2000), and since they do not always agree with how physicians and hospitals have integrated it. This shows that social movement outcomes are not always intended by activists (Clemens 1993, Glenn 1999), and that outcomes are more accurately thought of as a process rather than an end product (Einwohner 1999). This also illustrates that activists do not always agree on the goals a movement should pursue. While some activists welcome integration, others prefer separation. 'Hence a given change is not necessarily perceived as a success by all sectors of a movement' (Giugni 1999: xx).

I merge social movement and institutional theories to understand how social movements and institutions interact dynamically. Social movement theorists rarely study how elites in social institutions, such as medicine, respond to movements (Giugni 1998, 1999, Moore 1999). Institutional theories overcome this limitation by showing how social institutions respond to external demands. Institutional theory also limits our understanding of this dynamic relationship, because theorists infrequently examine how social movements demand changes of established organisations. Social movement theories illuminate this relationship from the perspective of activists. Merging these two theories brings a fuller understanding of how Western medicine responds to the CAM movement, and how activists respond in turn. After reviewing the social movement and institutional literature and describing my methods, I provide evidence of how Western medicine responds to the CAM movement and how activists perceive each response.

Institutional theories

Institutional theories examine how mainstream organisations respond to pressures to change; researchers, however, have criticised theorists for ignoring the role of agency and organisational self-interest (Chaves 1996, Oliver 1991, Zucker 1991). As government, professions, interest groups or public opinion exert pressure on organisations, early institutional theorists implied that organisations adapt accordingly. An organisation co-opts or 'absorbs new elements into their leadership or policy' to win their consent, power or resources, as when the Tennessee Valley Authority allowed outside constituencies to modify its programmes in exchange for their preservation (Selznick 1949: 34). Pfeffer and Salancik (1978: 167) argue that organisations co-opt interest groups that are 'politically potent'. 'New' institutional theories suggest that established organisational fields are homogeneous because each organisation has to concede to environmental pressure to remain stable (Meyer and Rowan 1977); thus they mimic others they deem successful (DiMaggio and Powell 1983). Actors comply since the gains, especially organisational stability in the face of intense competition, usually outweigh any required modifications (Perrow 1972, Scott 1987, Shortell *et al.* 1990). This is why 'fringe' players cannot only force organisational change, but institutionalise their innovations (Leblebici *et al.* 1991: 358–9).

Later institutional theorists view organisations as more active players. I focus on Oliver's (1991) work since she provides such a thorough range of possible responses. She argues that organisations can avoid, acquiesce to, compromise with, manipulate, or defy external demands. Organisations can *avoid* changing by concealing their noncompliance. Meyer and Rowan (1977) show that some organisations only symbolically accept institutional requirements while being publicly inspected; thereby, concealing their nonconformity. *Acquiescence* is the most passive response because organisations simply accede to external pressures. This includes the imitation process outlined by DiMaggio and Powell (1983). With *compromise*, organisations conform to the external constituents' demands, but with some resistance. Administrators may comply with a new governmental policy, but negotiate a reduction in the 'frequency or scope of its compliance' (Oliver 1991: 154). Organisations can *manipulate* the threat as Selznick (1949) describes within the Tennessee Valley Authority. Finally, *defiance* entails more active resistance such as dismissing or attacking a challenger. After some modification, I use her terms to argue that elites can avoid (avoidance), join (compromise), integrate (acquiescence), co-opt (manipulation) or counter (defiance) a social movement.

Institutional theories illustrate how social institutions such as medicine can respond in multiple ways to external demands, though theorists rarely examine social movements. I now turn to social movement theories to understand this relationship from the activists' perspective.

Social movement theories

Social movement theorists increasingly describe social movement outcomes by focusing on activists, social movement organisations, institutions, public policy and larger culture[3], but most examine political outcomes (Giugni 1998, 1999, Moore 1999). This study focuses on elites to understand whether and how activists influence social institutions like medicine, because they control access to these mainstream institutions. Physicians and hospital administrators are an elite group in relation to the CAM movement, because they are gatekeepers to CAM's entry into Western medicine. Theorists have differing ideas on how much influence social movements can have and what role elites play in relation to movements.

Most social movement theorists examine how elites within political, rather than social, institutions respond to movements. Moore (1999), an exception, argues that social institutions are more vulnerable to protest than the government, because they 'have less ability to create and use law, and have little ability to use violence and repression to stifle dissent' (1999: 97). Social institutions are vulnerable when institutional actors have extensive autonomy as is the case with physicians (Freidson 1970a, 1970b). Social institutions can change the type of people allowed in the institution and what subjects the institution examines and how. In medicine 'protest may change who counts as a healer by including new groups or excluding others' (Moore 1999: 102). Changes typically occur in isolated areas rather than the entire institution.

Social movement theories illuminate the relationship between institutional actors and movements from the activists' perspective. Elites can avoid, assist, join, integrate, co-opt or counter a social movement, which is why activists have mixed feelings about these outcomes. First, elites can *avoid* activists' demands. The hospice movement established independent agencies, because hospitals were sceptical (Abel 1986). Second, elites may *assist* social movements by providing resources. Jenkins and Eckert (1986) show how private foundations funded civil rights movement organisations. Third, elites may *participate as activists*, pursuing movement goals through their work as scientists (Moore 1996, Walsh 1986), government officials (Eisenstein 1995, Ferree and Hess 1995, Halcli and Reger 1996), lawyers and physicians (Taylor 1996, Whittier 1995). These 'institutional activists' (Santoro and McGuire 1997) give movements legitimacy, and can serve as 'mediators' who 'translate the challenges of protesting groups' into institutions (Moore 1999: 113). Fourth, elites may *allow activists to join their organisation*. Government officials granted access to homeless activists (Cress and Snow 2000) and feminists (Ferree and Hess 1995), and hospitals incorporated hospice leaders (Abel 1986).

Fifth, elites can *co-opt* a movement. Resource mobilisation theorists McCarthy and Zald (1973, 1977) argue that elites will eventually co-opt social movement organisations[4]. Political process theorists warn that since elites have a vested interest in maintaining the status quo, they may try to restrain a movement's mobilisation potential (Gamson 1968, Jenkins and Eckert 1986, Oberschall 1973) by forcing activists to pursue moderate goals or tactics by threatening to withdraw support (McAdam 1982, McCarthy and Zald 1987, Meyer 1993). In Gamson's (1990) model, co-optation means that a movement has gained acceptance without advantages such as policy changes. Garner (1996: 35) suggests that institutions co-opt activists by allowing them insider status, but restricting their work to 'a limited set of reforms'. Hospitals employed hospice leaders, but rather than instituting a team approach, they were subjected to physician supervision (Abel 1986). Informal co-optation occurs when elites facilitate a movement, but do not grant activists formal institutional access (Kriesi *et al.* 1992). Some hospitals used hospice ideas, but did not hire activists (Abel 1986). Activists often view co-optation negatively; however, Paul *et al.* (1997) argue that some goals are partially realised.

Finally, elites can *constrain* a movement. Countermovements have formed against movements for women (Ferree and Hess 1995), civil rights (Barkan 1984, McAdam 1983, Parker 1990), the environment (van der Heijden 1997), animal rights (Jasper and Poulsen 1993), labour (Fantasia 1988, Griffin *et al.* 1986) and the poor (Piven and Cloward 1977, Weyland 1995). Counter-movements arise when a movement achieves some level of success, which makes some group feel threatened (Meyer and Staggenborg 1996).

Combining institutional and social movement theories enables us to examine the outcomes of the CAM movement. Institutional theories have studied social institutions more extensively than social movement theorists. Yet, the social movement literature shows how institutional actors respond to activists, because the institutional literature has rarely examined how social movements demand institutional changes.

Data and methods

I used two data sources to examine the relationship between movements and institutional actors. The first examined Western medicine's view of CAM. I administered a phone survey of hospitals in Boston, Massachusetts and the Capital District of New York to see whether they offered CAM. I asked to speak with a hospital representative who was familiar with their services, and this person varied from hospital to hospital. To examine how hospitals integrate CAM, I then arranged semi-structured interviews with seven people representing two hospitals in Boston and four hospitals in the Capital District that all offered CAM. There were four nurses, one physician and one occupational therapist; however, four of the seven were administrators.

The second source of data examined the San Francisco, California Bay area, because it is the centre of activity for the CAM movement (Baer *et al.* 1998, Berliner and Salmon 1979). I conducted semi-structured interviews with 30 alternative practitioners (including one physician and three nurses) and 10 consumers[5] about whether and how they identify as activists. I found most practitioners by examining the local telephone directory, and most clients by asking to speak to the practitioners' clients, posting fliers in clinics, and using snowball sampling. The majority of interviews were tape recorded. I also observed five organisations: a women's clinic, a solo practitioner, an integrative clinic, a professional association, comprising physicians and alternative practitioners exploring integrative medicine, and an interest group educating the public about CAM. I found these organisations through the telephone directory and word of mouth, and gained entrée by asking the director for permission to study the organisation.

I analysed the data[6] using inductive and deductive methods. I coded the data into broad categories like 'outcomes', and then identified themes within these categories, such as 'moderating discourse to gain entrée'. I drew theoretical conclusions within each category based on common themes that emerged. I used induction to derive most of the types of outcomes, but after reviewing Oliver's (1991) work, I used deduction to add other outcomes that were better represented by outside literature than by my data. All of the outcomes I found fitted into Oliver's categories. These data shed light on how institutional actors respond to the CAM movement even though they are limited by geography and number of physicians interviewed.

Next, I identify the five outcomes. Three sections (*i.e.* avoidance, compromise and defiance) use data from the Bay area sample since this is where I studied non-hospital settings; whereas, the remaining two sections (*i.e.* acquiescence and manipulation) are based on the Northeast sample, which uses hospital data.

Outcomes

I adapt Oliver's (1991) typology to explain the complexity of organisational responses to the CAM movement. Some physicians respond passively by ignoring activists' demands while others actively respond by developing integrative clinics with alternative practitioners. Administrators respond positively by hiring activists to work inside their hospitals, but they respond negatively by restricting their activities.

Avoidance
Oliver's (1991) version of avoidance includes symbolic changes that create the illusion of compliance; whereas, I modify this slightly to mean that the organisation does not change, and they do not feel any need to do so, even symbolically. Mainstream medicine avoided a more active, collective response to the CAM movement until the mid-1990s. Avoidance can take the form of a lack of services or knowledge. Eighty-four per cent of hospitals did not offer any alternative techniques in 2000 (www.aha.org). One massage therapist adds that 'doctors sometimes don't know what chiropractic work is all about'. The professional association's newsletter acknowledges that 'among both conventional and complementary professionals, there has been a tendency toward isolation and lack of awareness of how others work'.

Elites may still assist the challenger. This is similar to Kriesi *et al.*'s (1992) definition of informal co-optation, where a group does not gain formal access, but receives assistance. Assistance typically entails referrals. One alternative clinic 'refer[s] back and forth' with one physician. The director explains that 'we support each other in that way, [and] build those relationships'. One client knows 'doctors [who] will encourage people to pursue different things if they don't feel that it's going to be destructive, [but only until] their colleagues start kidding them about it'.

Three caveats are important, given that you would not expect any form of assistance with avoidance. First, individual elites, not established organisations, are assisting the challenger. Second, there is often no communication between these healthcare providers so there is more avoidance than alliance. Third, many physicians are reluctant to admit to colleagues that they make these referrals. One respondent finds that 'when I talk to MDs [medical doctors] . . . they almost feel that they have to be fairly quiet about what they are doing, for fear of censure by their own peers'. Another respondent believes physicians are afraid of malpractice suits. The discrete nature of their individual actions maintains the illusion of collective avoidance.

Consequently, when an organisation avoids the pressure to accommodate activists' demands, the challengers must remain as outsiders. Many activists continue to work through an alternative model (Clemens 1993). Avoidance is reflected in the term 'alternative medicine', which implies that techniques are practiced *outside* Western medicine. The majority of alternative practitioners in the Bay area had little contact with physicians. One Reiki practitioner said she 'never' discussed her work with physicians, because 'it wouldn't make any difference'. These alternative practitioners remain isolated from Western medicine despite the occasional referral. From this vantage point, a hypnotherapist stated, 'right now, it looks like [alternative medicine] will be distinct [from Western medicine]'. Another person training to be a naturopath explains, 'because it is an alternative type of medicine, you are on the fringe, and so you by default have to stick together'.

Avoidance becomes a less viable organisational response for Western medicine as more consumers try CAM. One respondent says it is now not a question of 'whether or not' CAM will be integrated into Western medicine, but 'how will it be done'. Compromise, in the form of integrative clinics, occurs outside Western medical settings; whereas, the remaining three responses take place inside hospitals, and follow Oliver's (1991) definitions more closely.

Compromise
Oliver's (1991) notion of compromise entails an established organisation conforming, but with some resistance. I change this to recognise that some insiders may leave their organisation because they find the opposition's ideas appealing. These institutional actors compromise by creating a hybrid organisation with the opposing group on more neutral ground. These activists are developing an organisational innovation new to the United States healthcare system in addition to forming a compromise between the alternative and Western models[7].

Integrative clinics are the best example of a compromise between alternative practitioners and physicians. The integrative clinic I studied comprised a physician, nurse, acupuncturist, homeopath, bodyworker, chiropractor, counsellor and hypnotherapist. Practitioners advertise under one collective name and act as a team even though they pay rent individually and do not share fees. A physician and homeopath first examine a client since, according to respondents, those fields are adept at diagnosing conditions. Then all practitioners work together to devise a treatment plan that includes various modalities. Someone with carpal tunnel syndrome may see the physician, movement re-educator and bodyworker for treatment. All techniques are practiced in accordance with holistic ideology.

One respondent suggests that 'for a while [the movement] didn't include many physicians and now that seems to be one of the groups that's leading the way'. Since this response reflects physicians' growing acceptance of CAM, it is important to understand why physicians would become more open to these techniques. Goldstein *et al.* (1987) found that, compared to family practice physicians in California, physicians in the American Holistic Medical Association were less likely to have attended a medical school in the United States. Goldstein *et al.* (1985) found that members of Physicians in Transition, a support group of holistically-oriented physicians, became interested because of increasing dissatisfaction with their Western practices, personal experience with illness that could not be treated with Western medicine to their satisfaction, and their involvement in social networks that advocated CAM.

This study cannot definitively say why physicians would explore CAM, but there are many possibilities that expand upon Goldstein's work. The first is that some may begin to explore alternatives because of structural changes within Western medicine, especially during the last 30 years, that have eroded physicians' autonomy and legitimacy (Goldner 2000). Ownership and control of hospitals has shifted to financial managers (Gray 1986, Scott and Backman 1990) who may question physicians' professional judgement or restrict their time with patients because of concern with profits (Scott 1993). One member of the professional association thinks that:

> managed care increases the frustration for MDs . . . they are under time restraints where they can't treat people. They just have to give a quick pill . . . they realise the side effects that go along with those, and they are unhappy with that.

As one physician in the professional association said, physicians are now 'on the outside', meaning that power has shifted to insurance companies, managed care and the government. He added that 'patients are complaining, [and] we are beginning to, as well'. One member noted that in the professional association 'there's a lot of dissatisfaction [with Western medicine], especially among allopathic doctors looking for changes'. Some may begin to explore alternatives outside Western medicine, especially if they are drawn to the ideology behind CAM.

A second possibility is that some physicians recognise the limits of Western medicine and the benefits of CAM. The integrative clinic's director explains that their practitioners, including the physician, recognised 'their limitations'. Respondents suggested that Western medicine was useful for diagnosing and monitoring conditions, as well as resolving acute crises such as broken bones, while CAM was better for treating chronic diseases. In their opinion a unification of Western medicine and CAM, or integrative medicine, is more beneficial than choosing either one exclusively. The clinic director said, 'I think a lot of these groups are forming to combine resources and cover more of the bases. We recognised that people need the whole spectrum [of resources] to get better and stay that way'. Their goal is to provide 'comprehensive healthcare that works better than any one approach by itself' (clinic flyer). One physician says this combination allows for an 'expanded selection of tools for helping my patients' (professional association's newsletter). Physicians may reach this conclusion as they begin to agree with holistic ideology that dictates a much broader focus on physical, spiritual and emotional healing.

Most physicians will not leave their hospitals to develop integrative clinics, so now I turn to their responses inside hospitals. Hospitals are affected by the same factors as previously mentioned, given that physicians are a leading force within hospitals and that managed care is forcing these institutions to cut costs. Yet, as will be seen in the next section, two additional factors explain why *more* physicians, and the hospitals where they work, are beginning to integrate CAM.

Acquiescence

An established organisation responds to activists when they believe the movement is an external threat or has a legitimate claim. The CAM movement posed a 'threat' by the growing numbers using CAM. The turning point came when Eisenberg *et al.* (1993, 1998) showed that more individuals were using CAM than previously thought (Cowley 2002, Wolpe 1999). One respondent said that physicians in the professional association 'quote Eisenberg a lot. That was [published] in the *New England Journal of Medicine*, and it's their premier journal'.

Yet, consumer usage was not enough for some physicians to advocate integration of CAM into Western medicine, because many were still concerned about its safety and efficacy. One occupational therapist said that physicians want scientific evidence before they offer these techniques in her hospital. The movement is 'legitimated' when the government finds enough merit in the challenger's stance for them to begin to investigate. The CAM movement gained legitimacy through funding from the National Institute of Health (NIH), which is channelled through the National Center for Complementary and Alternative Medicine (NCCAM). This research has increased the credibility of some forms of CAM even though much research remains. One hospital nurse said that she felt 'hopeful' that CAM was now:

tied into one of the NIH research centers . . . knowing that the government is investing some money into research legitimates [CAM] for a lot of the medical community or it can in the future. If it's legitimated, I think that that's where [integration is going to] come from, because I think that there's so much going on now, not that it's enormous but so much compared to the past, that as that continues to grow, it will be harder and harder to ignore that. So there won't be an article here and there. It will be larger and maybe that will generate some excitement and enthusiasm for people to look at it a little bit differently.

As the CAM movement becomes more visible, and especially as scientists gather more research on the safety and efficacy of specific techniques, mainstream organisations will respond more directly to the movement. Acquiescence is the most passive of these responses, because organisations simply accede to external pressures. Hospitals acquiesce or 'comply in anticipation of self-serving benefits', which could entail protection from public criticism or financial gain (Oliver 1991: 153). Increased legitimacy and usage have led to greater levels of insurance reimbursement (Edlin 2003, Lee and Ryan 2000), so hospitals may incorporate CAM to secure their market share. Managed care has also forced hospitals to cut costs, and CAM advocates suggest that these techniques are less costly.

Institutionalised actors acquiesce when they allow challengers to join their organisation and work toward movement goals. Alternative practitioners worked in all six hospitals I examined, and were able to practice their techniques in accordance with holistic beliefs. One hospital allowed alternative practitioners to stress the connection between the mind and the body and individual responsibility for health. At another hospital where they employ a music therapist, a hospital administrator said:

we believe in treating the whole person – body, mind, and spirit – and this includes families. Complementary therapies can empower patients and help them to regain some of the control that is lost when diagnosed [with a disease]. Our patients now have access to a whole array of services to treat their whole being.

This organisational response illustrates one version of complementary medicine, which entails using these techniques as adjuncts to Western medicine. Another version of complementary medicine entails manipulation.

Manipulation
Manipulation involves organisations trying to 'establish power and dominance over the external constituents [who] are applying pressure on the

organisation' (Oliver 1991: 158). Establishment leaders give the opponents access, but restrict their activities in some way. This fits Garner's (1996) and Gamson's (1990) definitions of co-optation. Organisations can also co-opt ideas, techniques or other innovations, without giving access to 'fringe players' (Leblebici *et al.* 1991: 359). Organisations manipulate the CAM movement by allowing alternative practitioners to work in their hospitals without using holistic ideology, or by incorporating the techniques of the movement but not the activists. The former entails co-optation of personnel, while the latter involves co-optation of ideas.

Co-optation of movement ideas is becoming more widespread. Almost two-thirds of medical schools now offer courses on CAM (Wetzel *et al.* 1998). One hospital occupational therapist said that physicians have been increasingly tolerant since the mid-1990s, because of a growing amount of information on CAM at medical conferences. Physicians manipulate CAM when they use these techniques on patients. An estimated 3,000 physicians practise acupuncture (Langone 1996: 40), and an estimated one-third of homeopaths are physicians or osteopaths (Dranov 1996: 96). Physicians with Kaiser Permanente in Vallejo, California have practiced acupuncture for over a decade (Pelletier *et al.* 1997, Russell 1996). Several respondents noted that physicians are entering their training programmes for techniques such as homeopathy and naturopathy.

Physicians and hospitals 'appropriate' CAM in this way for several reasons (Adams and Tovey 2000). First, an occupational therapist from one of the hospitals believes that some physicians are worried about losing patients to alternative practitioners. A member of the professional association says that 'power rests in people . . . [so] change will come when people demand it' (field notes). One physician said that people in his profession are more 'materialistic', so they become interested in CAM when 'the market demands'. A hospital nurse said, 'people are spending money outside the hospital for this. Why shouldn't they spend it here?' Physicians need to practise these techniques to secure this revenue. Second, physicians may fear liability. One hospital nurse said that:

> there is a little more . . . openness toward [CAM], simply because some liability issues have been raised . . . doctors better know [about interactions between herbs and prescription drugs]. Someone's going to get sued, and that's how this will come to be an acceptable practice.

These fears could motivate some physicians to learn these techniques themselves. Third, if physicians practise CAM then the techniques have more credibility. One hospital physician said that it makes an 'enormous difference' if physicians practise these techniques, rather than an alternative practitioner who 'will always be seen as an outsider'. This hospital's goal is to train physicians in these techniques.

Defiance

The most damaging response is when organisational actors engage in defiance by not only resisting organisational change, but attacking the opposition (Oliver 1991). One respondent noted that as you attempt to change Western medicine by incorporating the ideas and techniques of CAM, 'you will get resistance'. Defiance entails mainstream actors going on the offensive or challenging the CAM movement often as a countermovement (Meyer and Staggenborg 1996, Mottl 1980). One respondent finds that 'the AMA [American Medical Association] and Western doctors are very threatened by naturopaths and alternative practitioners. It's their livelihood that is being threatened'. One physician notes that historically:

> the AMA clearly . . . had an agenda to eliminate other forms of practice. Obviously, [the] AMA lost the famous Chiropractic litigation, but they . . . also consciously attacked Naturopathic, Homeopathic, etc[8].

Some respondents were still suspicious of the AMA even though they passed a resolution in 1995 encouraging more research and education on CAM. Some alternative practitioners spoke of state laws restricting their practices, and more importantly, the knowledge that physicians can 'restrict us whenever they want'. One respondent said that 'traditional medicine, probably the AMA [American Medical Association]', is behind legislation to increase the educational and training requirements for California hypnotherapists. She said:

> I know that chiropractors went through the same kind of thing several years back. Whenever a new specialty comes around that seems to be taking some of their clients, there is always a push for legislation.

Not all alternative practitioners are opposed to increased educational and training requirements, and many advocate this to increase their legitimacy. These activists would like to be behind such strategies, though, as opposed to groups such as the AMA.

Counter movements also attempt to restrict the movement's goals through scientific, not just political, strategies. The National Council Against Health Fraud (NCAHF) is a non-profit agency concerned with 'health fraud, misinformation and quackery' (www.ncahf.org). The NCAHF says that acupuncture is 'based on primitive and fanciful concepts of health and disease that bear no relationship to present scientific knowledge; research during the past twenty years has failed to demonstrate that acupuncture is effective against any disease' (www.ncahf.org). To protect consumers, this group desires more scientific evidence, education for physicians and restrictions on lay practitioners. Another group that has questioned the safety and efficacy of CAM is Quackbusters, founded in 1969 by Dr. Stephen Barrett. As one physician said, 'Quackbusters are the brown shirts of allopathic medicine'.

Activists' perception of outcomes

Activists react to each organisational response differently, given the lack of consensus within the movement. The terms alternative, complementary and integrative medicine reflect the differing goals within the movement. Alternative medicine implies complete separation from Western medicine. Consumers use these techniques as an alternative to Western medicine, and the practitioners are segregated from hospitals and physicians. A cancer patient may use massage and herbs in lieu of chemotherapy, for example. Complementary medicine entails using these techniques as adjuncts to Western medicine, but Western medicine remains the dominant modality. Here the cancer patient would use chemotherapy as the main treatment, but supplement with massage and herbs. Activists define integrative medicine as using both Western and alternative techniques while maintaining the ideology of CAM (*e.g.* the mind-body connection). Some activists desire integration while others do not. *Purists* want to create an alternative medical model, because they do not desire integration of any kind. *Mainstreamers* and *moderates*, two types of integrative activists, both want to interact with Western medicine, but in very different ways. Mainstreamers are content with complementary medicine while moderates insist on integrative medicine. I now describe activists' perceptions of these responses to illustrate this heterogeneity and to understand the dynamic relationship between the movement and established actors.

Avoidance

Elites' avoidance has isolated many activists, but activists differ as to whether this is positive or negative. Purists do not desire any contact with physicians, because they do not want to lose their independence as practitioners, or they do not see the value of Western medicine as consumers. One activist said, 'both sides are weary of the other'. An acupuncturist notes that 'Western medicine has nothing to offer or what they have to offer is dangerous'. Most activists are not content to remain as outsiders, because they value Western techniques. One homeopath said he 'recognised that there had to be bridges built . . . with the mainstream'. Their desire for integration is also strategic, because they gain credibility through integration. Western medicine's avoidance leads to blocked opportunities, but many activists respond by seeking physician allies (Weyland 1995). Mainstreamers and moderates differ in the types of interactions they prefer with physicians.

Compromise

Elites' use of compromise has encouraged many integrative activists, because of the equality between practitioners and the retention of beliefs. Physicians and nurses are practising Western medicine, so alternative practitioners maintain control over their techniques; all practitioners, however, are using their techniques in accordance with holistic beliefs. According to respondents, alternative practitioners need equal power for integrative medicine to work. Though integrative medicine can be practised in a hospital, this equality is more likely to occur on neutral terrain since hospitals are physician-centred models. Yet, one practitioner said the physician still threw her weight around in the integrative clinic. Practitioners also had difficulty learning how to communicate with such diverse world views and languages, and figuring out how to obtain insurance reimbursement for all services so that patients truly had options. Given the importance of holistic beliefs, which will be discussed later, integrative activists still thought highly of this model despite these difficulties.

Acquiescence
Activists have disparate reactions when elites acquiesce to the movement. On the one hand, acquiescence is positively regarded by moderates and main-streamers, because it entails diffusion of movement ideas and personnel within Western medicine. The significance of this will become clear as activists compare this to the next organisational response. On the other hand, 'access . . . is not influence' (Meyer 1993: 175), because acquiescence typically does not involve true integration of CAM. In one hospital:

> these techniques are practised within our disease centres on the clinic floors. Patients who choose to have Reiki receive it next door to someone receiving an infusion. We do not have a separate centre, because we want [CAM] to be truly integrated into our conventional services.

This is the exception, as many hospitals keep CAM separate from the rest of the hospital. In one hospital, alternative practitioners were allowed to teach classes on massage and hypnotherapy in an off-site clinic as independent contractors. Separation limits the beneficial impact that CAM can have, because alternative practitioners have varying abilities to influence their new co-workers. Physicians may not even know these services are offered. I had difficulty completing the hospital phone survey, because staff were not familiar with the forms of CAM offered in their hospitals. One hospital staff member admitted that most hospital staff do not know that these techniques are offered.

Even when physicians know of these services, alternative practitioners may still have difficulties influencing the hospital. One occupational therapist said that physicians like to keep CAM separate from what they do, and is not convinced that physicians want to 'integrate' these techniques into the hospital. She explains that physicians are 'hesitant' of some techniques, especially those that 'lack scientific background'. So even though this hospital educates the staff about CAM, and physicians have to write orders for some of these techniques, she believes that CAM is having a limited impact. In another hospital, one nurse felt as if there was not 'outright hostility' to her use of CAM, but at the same time she did not always receive as much support as she desired. She said 'they think it's just a gimmick, a distraction. Sure, if she wants to do that, fine. Let her'. In another hospital, a nurse said that she could not get physicians to discuss or refer patients for guided imagery. She said that physicians are already:

> experiencing enormous turmoil and change . . . [CAM] is just one more thing for them to pay attention to . . . you have to pick and choose very carefully what you put your time into . . . so why would you put it into something that is quirky?

Integrative activists do not push harder for integration, because they feel the need, as another nurse said, to 'go inch by inch. You don't want to bite the hand that feeds you'.

Manipulation

When physicians practice CAM, most activists feel it is a form of manipulation, because alternative practitioners have lost control of their techniques and ideology. One respondent said that 'acupuncturists are threatened by [a health maintenance organisation] training MDs to do this technique' in their clinics. There are at least three reasons why alternative practitioners are threatened by this practice, and why they perceive it as manipulation. First, physicians need 200 hours of training to practice acupuncture while a lay person needs 2,400 hours of clinical training and experience (Phalen 1998). One acupuncturist doubted that someone could learn the theory behind these practices in such a short time. He said 'they wouldn't let me do needle biopsy' after reading a book on the subject. Thus, 'MDs can practice acupuncture legally, but not well'. He believed that physicians 'won't get the same results, and you will get dissatisfied patients'. Acupuncturists in this study fear that the resulting patient dissatisfaction may reflect negatively on all acupuncturists.

Second, some physicians use alternative techniques without the underlying principles, because this would require more substantial changes in the way they practice. One physician interviewed said that only a 'minority of MDs want a different way to practice medicine'. A physician may practice acupuncture, but not stress the connections between the mind and the body. Physicians separate the technique from the beliefs, because it is time consuming (thus costly) for them to practice these techniques within the context of alternative beliefs. It takes more time for an acupuncturist to ask a patient about his or her wellbeing and teach this patient about lifestyle changes, than it does to insert acupuncture needles. One respondent knew of an acupuncturist who stopped training someone for this reason. This student was:

> abbreviating his training to incorporate it into [a HMO (Health Maintenance Organization). This HMO] accepts anything as reasonable as long as you can see six clients in an hour. That's where it goes awry.

He also fears that physicians may simply 'use herbs like prescription drugs'. They will be 'ineffective', because he believes that herbs are only effective if used in accordance with alternative principles. Some physicians do follow holistic ideology, and alternative practitioners could also separate the techniques from the beliefs. According to activists, this is less likely because alternative practitioners learn these beliefs when they learn the techniques, while physicians do not necessarily learn the beliefs, especially in the short training courses described above.

Finally, this type of co-optation is particularly difficult for activists to accept, because it confines them to a 'bitter role', as one acupuncturist put it, since they 'aren't part of it' when Western medicine and CAM merge. Physicians and insurance companies 'get all the glory and control' (and financial compensation) even though activists have done all the work. Another respondent adds that 'there's a certain amount of fear by alternative practitioners that MDs will co-opt what they have, since MDs already have the credibility and following. I think it's very possible'. The opposition receives credit for the movement's ideas at the same time that they exclude activists from the process of change. This follows Rochon's (1998: 196) argument that as the larger culture adopts a movement's ideas, non-activists can 'begin to portray themselves (and to be accepted by the media) as "experts" on the issue'. A movement may then 'lose control of its message, and correspondingly of the capacity to claim credit' (Meyer 2000: online). These issues are more of a concern for purists and moderates than mainstreamers.

Defiance
All types of activists spend time and resources responding to various forms of defiance or 'backlash', as one respondent put it. The interest group, in particular, lobbies politicians to ensure that individuals have the right to use and practice CAM. It is the movement's success that leads to the mobilisation of a countermovement, because it threatens elites' interests (Meyer and Staggenborg 1996, Weyland 1995).

Conclusion

Physicians and hospitals have begun to respond to the CAM movement given its popularity, but activists do not approve of all these organisational responses. Given the diversity of opinions on CAM, physicians avoid, compromise with, acquiesce to, manipulate or defy the demands of activists. Western medicine does not respond to the movement under *avoidance*, while *compromise* entails some physicians leaving Western medicine to form integrative clinics with alternative practitioners. Inside hospitals, alternative practitioners are allowed to work freely (*acquiescence*) or they are restricted in some way, or their ideas are co-opted (*manipulation*). Some institutional actors work against the movement through *defiance*. Just as institutional

actors respond in multiple ways, activists disagree as to whether these outcomes are favourable, given their differing goals. Activists who desire integration with Western medicine (*integrative activists*) prefer compromise and
acquiescence, and given the likelihood of defiance or manipulation, activists
who wish to remain separate from Western medicine (*alternative activists*)
prefer avoidance. Consequently, activists continually try to re-shape these
organisational responses, which means that these outcomes are continually
in process. The model proposed here expands upon institutional and social
movement theories, and may be applied to other movements.

This study adds empirical data to Oliver's (1991) theoretical framework,
and expands institutional theory. Institutional theorists have been *less* likely
to examine how organisations respond to social movements or contentious
politics according to McAdam and Scott (2002). This study shows how
activists perceive organisational responses both positively and negatively,
and consequently how outsiders engage in ongoing attempts to shape these
responses. This process of negotiation has led to newer organisational forms
such as integrative clinics or CAM centres within hospitals. This study illuminates emerging forms since institutional theory primarily examines existing forms and structures (McAdam and Scott 2002). 'Institutionalisation
does not bring us to a fixed point; it is, rather, a continuing and continually
challenged process' (Rootes 1999: 11). The same can be said for outcomes
more generally.

This study also expands social movement theory. First, Moore (1999) and
Giugni (1998, 1999) argue that few social movement theorists have examined
social institutions such as medicine. This study confirms Moore's (1999)
insights into social institutions such as that activists only impacted on isolated parts of the hospital since their work was kept separate. Even though
health movements have been studied by researchers in medical sociology and
science studies, Brown *et al.* (2004) point out that *social movement theorists*
have been less likely to study these movements[9]. They argue that health
movements move 'fluidly between lay and expert identities' or blur the distinction between insiders and outsiders (2004: 18). This expands our understanding of movement vs. institutional actors, because my study shows that
institutional actors can become activists and activists can become insiders.
Second, this study shows how institutionalised actors can control whether
and how they respond to activists' demands. It is inaccurate and incomplete
to view institutionalisation as 'simply present or absent'; rather, there are
different degrees (Zucker 1991: 83). Acquiescence is a different level of institutionalisation from manipulation. Though both entail integration of movement ideas, acquiescence also entails integration of activists. This argument
also recognises that elites respond differently to the same movement. Rather
than trying to answer whether a movement has been institutionalised or
not, as some have done, scholars need to ask how movements interact with
different organisations. Researchers must recognise these different levels of
institutionalisation before they can explain them.

Third, this study illustrates how activists perceive outcomes and resist co-optation. Many theorists assume that co-optation is a sign of failure; some activists, however, believe it is a sign of success. This study shows how activists interpret outcomes differently. Institutionalisation can equal success and failure (Meyer 1993), but it does not necessarily translate to co-optation. Activists believe that the strength and persistence of a movement's ideology should militate against co-optation of a movement's personnel and techniques (Goldner 2000). This argument has implications for researchers who study other social movements, because all movements interact in some way with the institutions they seek to change. Feminists have worked within the Catholic church (Katzenstein 1995), government (Eisenstein 1995, Spalter-Roth and Schreiber 1995) and academia (Whittier 1995) while AIDS, pro-choice and hospice activists have also gained institutionalised access (Abel 1986, Epstein 1996, Staggenborg 1991). Though some of these studies suggest that social movements do not necessarily become more conservative when they 'engage' established institutions (Reinelt 1995), many focus on co-optation as the end result (Abel 1986, DeFriese *et al.* 1989, DeVries 1984). Applying my model to their work could illustrate how established organisations respond to social movements in multiple ways, and whether activists have been able to use their ideology to resist co-optation. If established actors are interested in movement ideology, they are more likely to compromise or acquiesce; whereas, they are more likely to manipulate or defy activists if they only see the movement as a competitor.

A combination of social movement and institutional theories enables us to understand the dynamic relationship between the CAM movement and Western medicine since both lay people and experts are involved (Brown *et al.* 2004, Hess 2002). McAdam and Scott (2002) argue that these theorists should collaborate more:

> The so-called 'established' arenas – whether entire societies or sectors such as healthcare services – can undergo fundamental change, as prevailing conventions are questioned and entrenched interests challenged. In such situations, attending to the structure and actions of both established and emergent players is critical to understanding subsequent processes and outcomes (2002: 13).

My effort to link these two theories follows the precedent set by Clemens (1993) who describes how movements use multiple organisational forms and organisational insiders to achieve institutional change and resist co-optation, and Broad and Jenness (1996) who find that institutionalisation is an 'unfinished process' as DiMaggio (1989) claimed.

Future research should proceed in numerous directions to illuminate the dynamic relationship between this movement and the institutions it seeks to change. First, this trend is developing so rapidly that some responses will become more salient than others. Only a longitudinal, national study can detect how institutional actors respond differently over time and across the country, as well as what level of integration the CAM movement ultimately achieves with Western medicine. Despite the earlier and greater successes that the movement experienced in the San Francisco Bay area, this study shows that hospitals are integrating CAM in other areas. Researchers need to see if this trend continues. Since I examined California, New York and Massachusetts, this study cannot show how the movement is developing in other regions, but there should be regional differences. As Abbott (1991) argues, professionalization may follow different paths at the local, state and national level. Any future policy needs to recognise geographical differences.

Second, researchers should gather more data on hospitals and among physicians. This study combined their responses, because it examined the clinical response to CAM; however, these two institutional actors may begin to diverge in their responses, so it is critical to examine how they respond separately. Do hospitals respond in different ways because of location, leadership, size or strength of the local movement? More data are needed to see how individual physicians view CAM since this study is limited in the number of physicians interviewed. Is there a similar typology of physicians who are purists, mainstreamers and moderates, though these purists would only advocate Western medicine? How do various institutional actors respond to *specific* techniques? This study was concerned with how physicians and hospitals responded to *all* forms of CAM; future research, however, can begin to differentiate among CAM practices now that we have more examples of integration.

An acupuncturist believes that chiropractors are more 'adversarial' with Western medicine, because the American Medical Association 'acted aggressively against their work'. Chiropractors had to take the AMA to court to assert their right to practise (Cant and Sharma 2000). A client adds that his physician 'didn't think much of chiropractors'. There was less opposition among British physicians since chiropractors were seeking a 'more limited scope of chiropractic practice', which 'meant that it did not constitute a threat to the overall position of medicine, as it had done in the United States' (Cant and Sharma 2000: 432). Avoidance and defiance may be more likely than manipulation or acquiescence given chiropractor's stance historically in the US. Wardwell (1994), Goldstein *et al.* (1985) and Wolpe (1985) argue that physicians have already co-opted (or manipulated) acupuncture. This may result from the ease and speed with which one can learn the technique and the extent to which the technique can be separated from holistic ideology. The differing acceptance of various modalities should also be influenced by the amount of consumer usage (thus competition), scientific evidence supporting its safety and efficacy, licensing and educational standards and insurance reimbursement. Professionalization will also be affected by the amount of associations, organisational structures and professional knowledge that alternative practitioners create (Abbott 1991). Public policies need to acknowledge the diversity among CAM practices, and address specific techniques. Supporting this, the editors of the *New England Journal of Medicine* stated:

> there cannot be two kinds of medicine – conventional and alternative. There is only medicine that has been adequately tested and medicine that has not . . . Once a treatment has been tested rigorously, it no longer matters whether it was considered alternative at the outset. If it is found to be reasonably safe and effective, it will be accepted (Angell and Kassirer 1998: 841).

Third, future research should examine how other institutions respond, because professionalization takes place in a complex environment with multiple influences (Abbott 1988, 1998). For example, if the government recognises some techniques as a profession, this legitimacy would override much defiance against it, because 'it is ultimately the state which sanctions the degree of security and autonomy which a profession can enjoy' (Sharma 1992: 119). According to their professional organisations and the National Center for Complementary and Alternative Medicine, chiropractors are licensed in 50 states, acupuncturists in 40, massage therapists in 25 and naturopaths in 12. Professionalism could protect these practitioners from manipulation, but Astin *et al.* (1998) found that 19 per cent of physicians practised massage and chiropractic, and 17 per cent offered acupuncture. Avoidance and defiance may still be *more* likely than manipulation for chiropractic, especially given 'the tension between the collective stance and the individual practice of doctors' (Cant and Sharma 2000: 432). Cross-cultural research is important for understanding how the government influences the development of CAM. Since the United States is the only industrialised country without national health insurance, one would expect that the government has *less* of an influence in the US than other countries such as England.

Instead, the insurance industry plays a vital role in the US, which is why it is also important to study how insurers and managed care organisations are responding to CAM given that their policies control patients' access (Goldner 2001). Most patients in the integrative clinic could only use techniques that were reimbursed by insurance even when practitioners thought they should use additional modalities. This study does not examine how managed care and insurers respond to CAM, because it explores the clinical response to the movement; however, this is not an indication that their responses are not critical to the development of the movement, especially since they are increasingly reimbursing these techniques (Lee and Ryan 2001). Washington State passed a law in 1996 that requires reimbursement for alternative practices (Edlin 2003). Does this increase access for consumers, and can insurers meet the costs? Are these techniques more cost-effective, as proponents suggest?

Fourth, researchers need more data from the activists' perspective to capture the ongoing nature of outcomes. How do activists negotiate being both an insider and outsider (Epstein 1996)? Do alternative practitioners continue to identify as activists once inside hospitals, and do physicians who advocate CAM start to identify as activists? My research suggests that the movement will not disband simply because activists have gained institutional access; rather, they will continue to shape organisational responses. Yet, how does gaining institutional access blur the boundary between movements and mainstream organisations, and how does this ultimately impact upon the movement? Scholars can follow the lead of Moore (1999), Katzenstein (1995) and Epstein (1996). Policy makers need to include activists in their discussions since their views often differ from those of institutional actors.

It will take several years before we see how CAM and integrative medicine develop. Over time, more outcomes are certainly possible than the typology provided here. Whether and how consumers have access to these services is dependent on the dynamic relationship between Western medicine and the CAM movement, and on the heterogeneity within each group. As Wolpe (1999: 11) notes, 'even as biomedicine has fought alternatives it has nurtured them, drawn from them, used them as testing grounds. Even as alternatives have fought against the orthodoxy they have envied it, drawn from it, longed for legitimacy from it'.

Notes

1   This study focuses on the current CAM movement, which began in the late 1960s and early 1970s, even though physicians have accepted and rejected different forms of CAM since the 1800s.
2   Institutionalisation is 'the process by which a given set of units and a pattern of activities come to be normatively and cognitively held in place, and practically taken for granted as lawful (whether as a matter of formal law, custom, or knowledge)' (Meyer *et al.* 1987: 13).
3   See Giugni (1998) for a more complete review of the literature on social movement outcomes.
4   This is why Lowenberg argues that some theorists in the resource mobilisation tradition view co-optation as an inevitable, but 'one-directional linear model of change' (1989: 232–3).
5   Two were training to become alternative practitioners.
6   I did not use a computer package to analyse the data.
7   I borrow the term organisational innovation from the 'new institutionalism' literature, but modify it slightly to mean the creation of a new organisational form, rather than the diffusion of an innovation into existing organisations (Chaves 1996, Scott and Meyer 1994).
8   In the 1980s courts across the United States found that the AMA was in violation of the Sherman Antitrust law for trying to restrict referrals to chiropractors. Langone suggests that the AMA is 'the alternatives' chief antagonist' (1996: 42).
9   Notable exceptions include Brown's (1990) work on environmental health movements, Taylor's (1996) work on the post-partum depression movement and Ruzek's (1978) work on women's health movements.

References

Abbott, A. (1988) *The System of Professions*. Chicago: University of Chicago Press.

Abbott, A. (1991) The order of professionalization, *Work and Occupations*, 18, 355–84.

Abbott, A. (1998) Professionalism and the future of librarianship, *Library Trends*, 46, 430–44.

Abel, E.K. (1986) The hospice movement: institutionalizing innovation, *International Journal of Health Services*, 16, 71–85.

Adams, J. and Tovey, P. (2000) Complementary medicine and primary care: towards a grassroots focus. In Tovey, P. (ed.) *Contemporary Primary Care: the Challenges of Change*. Buckingham: Open University Press.

Angell, M. and Kassirer, J.P. (1998) Alternative medicine – the risks of untested and unregulated remedies, *New England Journal of Medicine*, 339, 839–41.

Astin, J.A., Marie, A., Pelletier, K.R., Hansen, E. and Haskell, W.L. (1998) A review of the incorporation of complementary and alternative medicine by mainstream physicians, *Archives of Internal Medicine*, 158, 2303–10.

Baer, H.A., Hays, J., McClendon, N., McGoldrick, N. and Vespucci, R. (1998) The holistic health movement in the San Francisco Bay area: some preliminary observations, *Social Science and Medicine*, 47, 1495–501.

Barkan, S.E. (1984) Legal control of the southern civil rights movement, *American Sociological Review*, 49, 552–65.

Berliner, H.S. and Salmon, J.W. (1979) The holistic health movement and scientific medicine: the naked and the dead, *Socialist Review*, 9, 31–52.

Broad, K.L. and Jenness, V. (1996) The institutionalizing work of contemporary antiviolence against women campaigns in the United States, *Research in Social Movements, Conflict and Change*, 19, 75–123.

Brown, P. and Mikkelsen, E. (1990) *No Safe Place: Toxic Waste, Leukemia, and Community Action*. Berkeley: University of California Press.

Brown, P., Zavestoski, S., McCormick, S., Mayer, B., Morello-Frosch, R. and Gasior, R. (2004) Health social movements: uncharted territory in social movement research, *Sociology of Health and Illness*, 26, 1–31.

Cant, S. and Sharma, U. (2000) Alternative health practices and systems. In Albrecht, G.L., Fitzpatrick, R. and Scrimshaw, S.C. (eds) *Handbook of Social Studies in Health and Medicine*. London: Sage Publications.

Chaves, M. (1996) Ordaining women: the diffusion of an organizational innovation, *American Journal of Sociology*, 101, 840–73.

Clemens, E. (1993) Organizational repertoires and institutional change: women's groups and the transformation of U.S. politics, 1890–1920, *American Journal of Sociology*, 98, 755–98.

Cowley, G. (2002) Now, 'integrative' care, *Newsweek*, 2 December, 46–53.

Cress, D.M. and Snow, D.A. (2000) The outcomes of homeless mobilization: the influence of organization, disruption, political mediation, and framing, *The American Journal of Sociology*, 105, 1063–104.

DeFriese, G.H., Woomert, A., Guild, P.A., Steckler, A.B. and Konrad, T.R. (1989) From activated patient to pacified activist: a study of the self-care movement in the United States, *Social Science and Medicine*, 29, 195–204.

DeVries, R.G. (1984) 'Humanizing' childbirth: the discovery and implementation of bonding theory, *International Journal of Health Services*, 14, 89–104.

DiMaggio, P.J. (1989) Interest and agency in institutional theory. In Zucker, L.G. (ed.) *Institutional Patterns and Organizations*. Cambridge, MA: Ballinger.

DiMaggio, P.J. and Powell, W.W. (1983) The iron cage revisited: institutional isomorphism and collective rationality in organizational fields, *American Sociological Review*, 48, 147–60.

Dranov, P. (1996) Alternative medicine: what helps, what hurts, *Ladies Home Journal*, November, 94–9.

Edlin, M. (2003) Demand for CAM grows, but belongs in separate benefit category, *Managed Healthcare Executive*, 13, 38.

Einwohner, R. (1999) Gender, class, and social movement outcomes: identity and effectiveness in two animal rights campaigns, *Gender and Society*, 13, 56–76.

Eisenberg, D.M., Kessler, R.C., Foster, C., Norlock, F.E., Calkins, D.R. and Delbanco, T.L. (1993) Unconventional medicine in the United States: prevalence, costs, and patterns of use, *New England Journal of Medicine*, 328, 246–52.

Eisenberg, D.M., Davis, R.B., Ettner, S.L., Appel, S., Wilkey, S., Van Rompay, M. and Kessler, R.C. (1998) Trends in alternative medicine use in the United States, 1990–1997: results of a follow-up national survey, *Journal of the American Medical Association*, 280, 1569–75.

Eisenstein, H. (1995) The Australian femocratic experiment: a feminist case for bureaucracy. In Ferree, M.M. and Martin, P.Y. (eds) *Feminist Organizations: Harvest of the New Women's Movement*. Philadelphia: Temple University Press.

Epstein, S. (1996) *Impure Science: AIDS, Activism, and the Politics of Knowledge*. Berkeley: University of California Press.

Fantasia, R. (1988) *Cultures of Solidarity: Consciousness, Action, and Contemporary American Workers*. Berkeley: University of California Press.

Ferree, M.M. and Hess, B. (1995) *Controversy and Coalition: the New Feminist Movement across Three Decades of Change*. New York: Twayne.

Freidson, E. (1970a) *Professional Dominance: the Social Structure of Medical Care*. New York: Atherton.

Freidson, E. (1970b) *Profession of Medicine: a Study of the Sociology of Applied Knowledge*. New York: Dodd, Mead.

Gamson, W. (1968) *Power and Discontent*. Homewood, IL: Dorsey.

Gamson, W. (1990/1975) *The Strategy of Social Protest*, 2nd Edition. Homewood, IL: Dorsey.

Garner, R. (1996) *Contemporary Movements and Ideologies*. New York: McGraw-Hill, Inc.

Giugni, M.G. (1998) Was it worth the effort? The outcomes and consequences of social movements, *Annual Review of Sociology*, 24, 371–93.

Giugni, M.G. (1999) How social movements matter: past research, present problems, future developments. In Giugni, M., McAdam, D. and Tilly, C. (eds) *How Social Movements Matter*. Minneapolis: University of Minnesota Press.

Glenn, J.K. (1999) Competing challengers and contested outcomes to state breakdown: the velvet revolution in Czechoslovakia, *Social Forces*, 78, 187–211.

Goldner, M. (1999) How alternative medicine is changing the way consumers and practitioners look at quality, planning of services and access in the United States, *Research in the Sociology of Health Care*, 16, 55–74.

Goldner, M. (2000) Integrative medicine: issues to consider in this emerging form of health care, *Research in the Sociology of Health Care*, 17, 213–33.

Goldner, M. (2001) Expanding political opportunities and changing collective identities in the complementary and alternative medicine movement, *Political Opportunities, Social Movements, and Democratization*, 23, 69–102.

Goldstein, M., Jaffe, D., Garell, D. and Berke, R.E. (1985) Holistic doctors: becoming a nontraditional medical practitioner, *Urban Life*, 14, 317–44.

Goldstein, M.S., Jaffe, D.T., Sutherland, C. and Wilson, J. (1987) Holistic physicians: implications for the study of the medical profession, *Journal of Health and Social Behavior*, 28, 103–19.

Gray, B. (ed.) (1986) *For-profit Enterprise in Health Care*. Washington, D.C.: National Academy Press.

Griffin, L.J., Wallace, M.E. and Rubin, B.A. (1986) Capitalist resistance to the organization of labor before the new deal: Why? How? Success? *American Sociological Review*, 51, 147–67.

Halcli, A. and Reger, J. (1996) Strangers in a strange land: the gendered experiences of women politicians in Britain and the United States. In Whittier, N., Taylor, V. and Richardson, L. (eds) *Feminist Frontiers*. New York, McGraw-Hill, Inc.

Hess, D.J. (2002) Technology-oriented social movements and the problem of globalization, Unpublished paper.

Jasper, J.M. and Poulsen, J. (1993) Fighting back: vulnerabilities, blunders, and countermobilization by the targets in three animal rights campaigns, *Sociological Forum*, 8, 639–57.

Jenkins, J.C. and Eckert, C.M. (1986) Channeling black insurgency: elite patronage and professional social movement organizations in the development of the black movement, *American Sociological Review*, 51, 812–29.

Katzenstein, M.F. (1995) Discursive politics and feminist activism in the Catholic Church. In Ferree, M.M. and Martin, P.Y. (eds) *Feminist Organizations: Harvest of the New Women's Movement*. Philadelphia: Temple University Press.

Kriesi, H., Koopmans, R., Duyvendak, J.W. and Giugni, M.G. (1992) New social movements and political opportunities in Western Europe, *European Journal of Political Research*, 22, 219–44.

Langone, J. (1996) Challenging the mainstream, *TIME Special Issue*, Fall, 40–3.

Leblebici, H., Salancik, G., Copay, A. and King, T. (1991) Institutional change and the transformation of interorganizational fields: an organizational history of the U.S. Radio Broadcasting Industry, *Administrative Science Quarterly*, 36, 333–63.

Lee, J. and Ryan, B. (2000) Easing the pain, *Money*, 29, 179–80.

Lowenberg, J. (1989) *Caring and Responsibility: the Crossroads Between Holistic Practice and Traditional Medicine*. Philadelphia: University of Pennsylvania Press.

McAdam, D. (1982) *Political Process and the Development of Black Insurgency, 1930–1970*. Chicago: University of Chicago Press.

McAdam, D. (1983) Tactical innovation and the pace of insurgency, *American Sociological Review*, 48, 735–54.

McAdam, D. and Scott, W.R. (2002) Organizations and movements. Paper presented at the Annual Meeting of the American Sociological Association, Chicago, IL.

McCarthy, J. and Zald, M. (1973) *The Trend of Social Movements in America*. Morristown, NJ: General Learning Press.

McCarthy, J. and Zald, M. (1977) Resource mobilization and social movements: a partial theory, *American Journal of Sociology*, 82, 1212–41.

McCarthy, J. and Zald, M. (1987) Resource mobilization and social movements: a partial theory. In Zald, M. and McCarthy, J. (eds) *Social Movements in an Organizational Society*. New Brunswick, NJ: Transaction Books.

Meyer, D.S. (1993) Institutionalizing dissent: the United States structure of political opportunity and the end of the nuclear freeze movement, *Sociological Forum*, 8, 157–79.

Meyer, D. (2000) Claiming credit: the social construction of movement success. (www.democ.uci.edu/democ/papers/meyer.htm).

Meyer, J. and Rowan, B. (1977) Institutionalized organizations: formal structure as myth and ceremony, *American Journal of Sociology*, 83, 340–63.

Meyer, J.W., Boli, J. and Thomas, G.M. (1987) Ontology and rationalization in the Western cultural account. In Thomas, G.M., Meyer, J.W., Ramirez, F.O. and Boli, J. (eds) *Institutional Structure*. Newbury Park, Sage.

Meyer, D. and Staggenborg, S. (1996) Movements, countermovements, and the structure of political opportunity, *American Journal of Sociology*, 101, 1628–60.

Moore, K. (1996) Organizing integrity: American science and the creation of public interest organizations, 1955–1975, *American Journal of Sociology*, 101, 1592–627.

Moore, K. (1999) Political protest and institutional change: the anti-Vietnam war movement and American science. In Giugni, M., McAdam, D. and Tilly, C. (eds) *How Social Movements Matter*. Minneapolis: University of Minnesota Press.

Mottl, T. (1980) The analysis of countermovements, *Social Problems*, 27, 620–35.

Oberschall, A. (1973) *Social Conflict and Social Movements*. Englewood Cliffs, New Jersey: Prentice-Hall.

Oliver, C. (1991) Strategic responses to institutional processes, *Academy of Management Review*, 16, 145–79.

Parker, F.R. (1990) *Black Votes Count: Political Empowerment in Mississippi after 1965*. Chapel Hill: The University of North Carolina Press.

Paul, S., Mahler, S.J. and Schwartz, M. (1997) Mass action and social structure, *Political Power and Social Theory*, 11, 45–99.

Pelletier, K.R., Marie, A., Krasner, M. and Haskell, W.L. (1997) Current trends in the integration and reimbursement of complementary and alternative medicine by managed care, insurance carriers, and hospital providers, *American Journal of Health Promotion*, 12, 112–23.

Perrow, C. (1972) *Complex Organizations: a Critical Essay*. Glenview, Illinois: Scott, Foresman and Company.

Pfeffer, J. and Salancik, G. (1978) *The External Control of Organizations: a Resource Dependence Perspective*. New York: Harper & Row, Publishers.

Phalen, K.F. (1998) *Integrative Medicine: Achieving Wellness Through the Best of Eastern and Western Medical Practices*. Boston: Journey Editions.

Piven, F. and Cloward, R. (1977) *Poor People's Movements*. New York: Vintage.

Reinelt, C. (1995) Moving onto the terrain of the state: the battered women's movement and the politics of engagement. In Ferree, M.M. and Martin, P.Y. (eds) *Feminist Organizations: Harvest of the New Women's Movement*. Philadelphia, Temple University Press.

Rochon, T.R. (1998) *Culture Moves*. Princeton: Princeton University Press.

Rootes, C. (1999) The transformation of environmental activism, *Innovation*, 12, 155–74.

Russell, S. (1996) HMOs try dose of alternative medicine, *San Francisco Chronicle*, January, A1, 4.

Ruzek, S.B. (1978) *The Women's Health Movement: Feminist Alternatives to Medical Control*. New York: Praeger.

Santoro, W. and McGuire, G. (1997) Social movement insiders: the impact of institutional activists on affirmative action and comparable worth policies, *Social Problems*, 44, 503–19.

Scott, R. (1987) The adolescence of institutional theory, *Administrative Science Quarterly*, 32, 493–511.

Scott, R. (1993) The organization of medical care services: toward an integrated theoretical model, *Medical Care Review*, 50, 271–302.

Scott, R. and Backman, E. (1990) Institutional theory and the medical care sector: early theory. In Mick, S. (ed.) *Innovations in Health Care Delivery: Insights for Organization Theory*. San Francisco: Jossey-Bass.

Scott, R. and Meyer, J. (1994) *Institutional Environments and Organizations: Structural Complexity and Individualism*. Thousand Oaks, California: Sage.

Selznick, P. (1949) *TVA and the Grass Roots*. Berkeley: University of California Press.

Selznick, P. (1948) Foundations of the theory of organization, *American Sociological Review*, 13, 25–35.

Sharma, U. (1992) *Complementary Medicine Today: Practitioners and Patients*. London: Tavistock/Routledge.

Shortell, S., Morrison, E. and Friedman, B. (1990) *Strategic Choices for America's Hospitals: Managing Change in Turbulent Times*. San Francisco: Jossey-Bass Publishers.

Spalter-Roth, R. and Schreiber, R. (1995) Outsider issues and insider tactics: strategic tensions in the women's policy network during the 1980s. In Ferree, M.M. and Martin, P.Y. (eds) *Feminist Organizations: Harvest of the New Women's Movement*. Philadelphia: Temple University Press.

Staggenborg, S. (1991) *The Pro-Choice Movement: Organization and Activism in the Abortion Conflict*. New York: Oxford University Press.

Taylor, V. (1996) *Rock-a-bye Baby: Feminism, Self-Help, and Postpartum Depression*. New York: Routledge.

TIME Special Issue (1996) *The Frontiers of Medicine*, Fall, 148.

van der Heijden, H. (1997) Political opportunity structure and the institutionalisation of the environmental movement, *Environmental Politics*, 6, 25–50.

Walsh, E.J. (1986) The role of target vulnerabilities in high-technology protest movements: the nuclear establishment at Three Mile Island, *Sociological Forum*, 1, 199–218.

Wardwell, W.I. (1994) Alternative medicine in the United States, *Social Science and Medicine*, 38, 1061–8.

Wetzel, M.S. (1998) Courses involving complementary and alternative medicine at US medical schools, *Journal of the American Medical Association*, 280, 784–7.

Weyland, K. (1995) Social movements and the state, *World Development*, 23, 1699–712.

Whittier, N. (1995) *Feminist Generations: the Persistence of the Radical Women's Movement*. Philadelphia: Temple University Press.

Wolpe, P. (1985). The maintenance of professional authority: acupuncture and the American physician, *Social Problems*, 32, 409–24.

Wolpe, P. (1999) From quackery to 'integrated care': power, politics, and alternative medicine, *Frontier Perspectives*, 10, 10–2.

Yoshida, M. (2002) A theoretical model of biomedical professionals' legitimization of alternative therapies, *Complementary Health Practice Review*, 7, 187–208.

Zucker, L. (1991) The role of institutionalization in cultural persistence. In Powell, W. and DiMaggio, P. (eds) *The New Institutionalism in Organizational Analysis*. Chicago, University of Chicago Press.

Chapter 4

Health consumer groups in the UK: a new social movement?

Judith Allsop, Kathryn Jones and Rob Baggott

Introduction

In the recent past, a number of new social movements across various countries have centred on struggles related to health and illness. A common factor in the genesis of these movements has been an individual experience of illness or bodily event which has led to identification with others in a similar position. Collective action occurs when people affected by a particular condition seek to alter the terms of engagement with healthcare providers and thus gain greater control over their own bodies. Some new social movements of the 1960s and 1970s concerned with health issues have been well documented. For example, various networks and groups related to maternity and childbirth grew out of the feminist movement (Lewin and Olesen 1985, Bastian 1998, Doyal 1998, Tew 1998). A mental health user movement also developed which grew from the experiences of those living with a mental illness, and aimed to represent their perspective (Brown 1984, Crossley 1999, Rogers and Pilgrim 2001). Similarly, movements related to disability (Campbell and Oliver 1996), HIV/AIDS (Epstein 1996, Weeks *et al.* 1996, Berridge 2002), gay and lesbian health (Weeks, Holland and Waites 2003) and health and environmental pollution (Brown *et al.* 2003) have developed from issues of concern to people in their everyday lives (Martin 2001).

This chapter aims to show, first, that the formation of networks and groups by people living with, or with experience of, a particular bodily condition has become more pervasive across a number of conditions. Such groups and networks have also formed in response to what Jennings (1999) terms 'pain and loss experiences': this broader category that includes not only illness, but a range of events that impinge on the bodily integrity of the self and others. Second, there is evidence of a shared discourse and values across the groups that promote and represent the interests of healthcare users. They promote lay knowledge and experience, and have contributed to the development of participative and consultative processes. This is true even for groups founded in an earlier period. Third, we suggest that as a consequence, collaboration between health consumer groups within the same condition area and across the sector, has increased to a degree where it is possible to point to a health consumer movement. Member groups provide the basis for collective action in the social and political sphere.

In investigating the formation of patient and carer groups, their relationships with each other, and their strategies for action, this chapter views such social groupings or movements as developing from personal experiences in the intimate and private aspects of life or, in the term used by Habermas (1984), 'the life world' of ordinary people. People are drawn into new social movements because they feel marginalised by dominant social practices, and movements gain adherents because a positive sense of identity can develop where perceptions are shared (Byrne 1997). Interaction both aids an individual in finding an explanation for a life event and helps to forge a collective identity through the development of a particular discourse and a set of perceptions and ideas on how action should be mobilised. Borkman (1999), in a study of groups in the United States, comments that self-help, mutual-aid groups and new social movements draw on narratives about personal experience to reconstruct negative identities and to plan action. As Rogers and Pilgrim (2001: 109) suggest in relation to mental health users, a particular identity is both 'a ticket to entry and a source of solidarity'.

This chapter also contributes to knowledge by showing that that there has been a 'spill-over effect' from earlier new social movements as newer groups draw on experience from the past and engage in the policy process and, thus, contribute to the politicisation of health issues (Melucci 1989, Meyer and Whittier 1994). Following Simon and Klandermans (2001), a broad definition of the political is taken. Groups become political when they approach third parties, and take action in the public arena. This may be concerned with obtaining redress, reshaping services, or by challenging the assumptions underlying policy and practice. A wider health consumer movement has the potential to shape services to make them more responsive to the concerns of patients and carers.

In making the arguments, the chapter draws on two research studies based in the United Kingdom (UK) undertaken by the authors. Data from the first, research on health consumer groups and their impact on the national policy process (called here the De Montfort study because it was conducted at De Montfort University) are drawn upon selectively and are reported on more fully elsewhere (Baggott, Allsop and Jones 2004). This is discussed in the first section of the chapter. We undertook the second study, the Protest Group study, to investigate health consumer groups largely excluded from the first study[1]. In this instance, groups had formed in response to adverse clinical events. We discuss the findings in the second section of the chapter together with an analysis of the differences between protest groups and general health consumer groups. The third section discusses the role of government in promoting the development of health consumer groups.

Health consumer groups in the UK

The De Montfort research aimed to study a cross-section of groups, their relationship with each other and their impact on the policy process at a national level. The term 'health consumer group' was used, rather than 'patient group'. This term was defined as: a voluntary sector organisation that seeks to promote and/or represent the interests of users and/or carers at national level, to capture experiences across a range of conditions, namely: arthritis, cancer, heart and circulatory disease, maternity and child-birth and mental health. Groups with interests across a range of conditions were also identified. Statutory organisations and research charities were excluded[2].

Research design and methods

We developed a questionnaire that aimed to map the characteristics and activities of groups: their internal structure, aims, activities and the type and frequency of contact with other organisations was developed. This was sent to the person within the group identified as being in charge of policy activity in the autumn of 1999[3]. The effective response rate was 66 per cent (123 groups). To aid the analysis we developed a typology of groups: 'condition-based groups' were defined as those focused on specific conditions and 'population-based groups' as those concerned with all patients, carers or a specific population sub-group, such as children or ethnic minorities across a range of conditions. 'Formal alliance organisations' were defined as groups made up of other autonomous groups but linked by a shared interest such as genetics or long-term illness[4]. SPSS was used to analyse the questionnaire data.

Subsequently, in 2000, we undertook semi-structured interviews with lead-ing members or paid officers from 39 health consumer groups. Although the interviews were with group leaders, not rank and file members, in practice these categories blurred. Those elected or appointed to leadership positions had been ordinary members; some were founder members. Interviewees who were employees, often had personal experience of conditions either directly or indirectly, and had been drawn to the sector for this reason. The interview sample reflected group characteristics such as size, type of group, condition area and date of formation. The interviews were taped, transcribed and entered into NVIVO qualitative data analysis software, and subsequently analysed to develop a grounded theory of internal and external dynamics. For the purposes of this chapter, we draw mainly on the dominant themes relating to the values and norms of groups, what interviewees saw as their 'expertise', and the internal processes of communication.

In the final stage of the research, semi-structured interviews were conducted with other policy actors and stakeholders (n = 31), including individuals from general consumer and research charities, professional organisations, the pharmaceutical industry and government. A fuller discus-sion of the research is available in a forthcoming book (Baggott, Allsop and Jones 2004).

Health consumer groups in the UK: characteristics

The groups identified in the research were extremely diverse. They had been formed at different times and according to different traditions. Some had

Table 1 *The date of formation of UK health consumer groups (De Montfort study)*

Date of formation	Percentage of Groups	Number of Groups
pre-1940	3	3
1941–1960	7	8
1961–1980	25	29
1981-date	66	77
Total	100	117*

Source: Questionnaire data set 1999
* data were missing for 6 groups
Due to rounding up, total exceeds 100

their origins in 19th-century philanthropy. Others had been established as charities in the post-second-world-war period to campaign for the extension of social rights, or had been set up for mutual support. Groups also varied considerably in size, in income and in their internal organisation. Larger groups sometimes had a structure of local branches while a few smaller groups, although their focus was country wide, were run from the home of a founder member.

Nevertheless, there were common characteristics. All groups, as might be expected, were concerned with issues related to illness, pain and loss. All focused on policy issues connected with the National Health Service (NHS), and none referred to private healthcare. Almost all groups were registered charities and over 90 per cent were membership groups, although in the mental health area there were a few charities that provided welfare services to clients on behalf of the state. Most groups prioritised a range of similar activities. These typically included providing information and advice for the general public, facilitating support services and activities for members, fundraising activities, raising awareness about a condition, and campaigning and lobbying on policy and services. Virtually all the groups were engaged in policy activity at a national level, although the scale of that activity and the tactics used, varied across different types of group depending on the policy context.

From the questionnaire data, Table 1 shows that two-thirds of health consumer groups in existence in 1999 had been formed in 1981 or after. This suggests an increase in the number of groups, a finding supported by Wood (2000) in his study of patient groups in Britain and the United States, although without a baseline date from which to measure it is not possible to be certain of the extent of this increase. More of the mental health groups had been established before 1981 (48%) than maternity and childbirth (40%) or arthritis (28%), heart and circulatory disease (23%) and cancer (22%) groups. Population-based groups (54%) were more likely to have been formed before 1981, while 68 per cent of condition-based groups and nearly three-quarters of formal alliance organisations (73%) were formed in 1981 or after.

Trends in group formation

Our interview data indicate that the formation of groups by people who have had personal experience of living with a condition has increased in recent years. Accounts of the formation of groups underline the findings of earlier studies that illness or bodily events bring a 'biographical disruption,' requiring a reconstruction of the self to take account of the changed status (Giddens 1979, Bury 1982, Charmaz 1983, and Williams 1984). Williams comments that narrative reconstructions can be used to 'reconstitute and repair ruptures between body, self and world by linking and interpreting different aspects of biography in order to realign present and past, self and society' (Williams 1984: 197). Williams comments that this may lead to various forms of action, but does not pursue the question of what leads people to form or join a group.

In the De Montfort research, common themes in the narratives of founder members of health consumer groups were: anger about what had happened to them; the perception that the condition was not well understood; a belief that service provision was inappropriate and a deep concern about the lack of information available for patients. Activists wanted to support others and to draw attention to shortcomings at a number of levels, such as changing the perceptions of professionals and the public and influencing national and local providers.

In terms of chronology, patient- or carer-led groups were formed first in the maternity and childbirth area or concerned children. Activists were mainly middle class, white women. In contrast, in the next wave – groups for mental health users – the social origins of activists were more mixed, although activists in the groups established by carers tended to be from the professional classes (Crossley 1999). In the literature and from our interviews, accounts illustrate the process through which others with similar views are identified and a group formed.

Within the maternity and childbirth sector, in the mid-1950s Prunella Briance established the National Childbirth Association. She had lost her baby and, attributing this to technological intervention, she founded the organisation in order to promote the use of gentler methods in childbirth (Tew 1998). Renamed in 1961 and with a membership of 45,000 and 450 branches nation-wide, the National Childbirth Trust (NCT) is now the largest maternity and childbirth consumer group in the UK. The NCT works with both local and national groups to put pressure on the national government to improve maternity services.

The Association for Improvements in the Maternity Services (AIMS) was formed in 1960 and, although initially set up simply to improve access to services, it has developed into a more radical group committed to increasing women's control over childbirth and, if they wish, to have a home birth.

AIMS has become highly critical of technological interventions, and a former activist commented on the shared identity of members saying: 'typically, they have become active after having their first child and they see themselves as having been assaulted' (group interview 42). The perpetrators in this instance were identified as 'OWMs', the 'old white men' of the medical profession – male obstetricians who at that time dominated the profession. AIMS was one of the few groups in the De Montfort study where interviewees believed that charity status would undermine their independence and their ability to be outspoken and critical.

An absence of support also triggered the formation of groups such as the Twins and Multiple Births Association (TAMBA) in 1978, which aims to help parents cope with a multiple birth, and the Stillbirth and Neonatal Death Society (SANDS) in 1981, formed by parents who had been devastated by a stillbirth. Members of both groups had used their own experience to provide support for others. Despite some differences in priorities and tactics, groups in the maternity sector now actively collaborate with each other: they share the same broad objectives; they have similar perceptions; they sympathise with the feminist movement and have struggled against the medicalisation of childbirth. Each group tends to occupy a particular niche, so they do not compete directly. In recent years, the interests of maternity groups and medical professionals have converged as maternity services have slipped down the Governments' policy agenda. Nevertheless, some groups collaborate with professional associations more actively than others.

Group formation following a personal experience is also apparent in the mental health field. Many groups have been established by carers, or have emerged out of carers' experiences. The National Schizophrenia Fellowship was established in 1972 by a carer who wrote about his experiences in the letters page of *The Times* newspaper and reached a wide audience of people in a similar position (Levy 1981). Schizophrenia a National Emergency (SANE), was formed in 1986 by Marjorie Wallace, a journalist who wrote an influential series of articles, also in *The Times*, about the care of people with schizophrenia. These brought to public attention the plight of sufferers and their families, and according to Rogers and Pilgrim (2001) SANE has been successful in keeping these issues on the policy agenda. In addition, service users have played a significant role in the formation of national groups such as Survivors Speak Out and the UK Advocacy Network (Rogers and Pilgrim 1991).

Most mental health groups are unified by a history of struggle against the power of the medical profession and a concern to respect the dignity, social rights and autonomy of people living with mental illness. There are exceptions, such as one group in the interview sample, the Zito Trust, formed in 1994 by Jayne Zito after the murder of her husband by a man with a severe mental illness who was receiving care in the community (Rogers and Pilgrim 2001). Unlike most other mental health groups, the Zito Trust campaigns on issues that give a higher priority to public safety than to the civil rights of those with mental health problems. This suggests that the politics of pain and loss are not necessarily emancipatory or progressive, but can stem from, and reflect, deeply-held fears supported by a body of public opinion. The British tabloid press gives widespread coverage to the perceived 'dangers' posed by people with a mental illness living in the community. One consequence is that other mental health groups have found common cause with progressive elements of the medical profession and have formed a broadly-based lobby group, the Mental Health Alliance.

In the 1980s and 1990s, several new cancer groups were established by those with direct experience of the disease as either patients or carers. For example, CancerBACUP was founded in 1985 by Vicky Clement-Jones who was diagnosed with ovarian cancer when in her early 30s. She was appalled by the lack of information available, and the charity is now dedicated to providing accurate and up-to-date information for patients and carers. As a doctor but not a cancer specialist, Clement-Jones worked closely with others living with the illness as well as with health professionals. On her death, her own oncologist took over as chair of the organisation (Clement-Jones 1985). Cancerlink (1982), the National Cancer Alliance (1994) and the UK Breast Cancer Coalition (1995) were also formed by young women affected by cancer to support others and campaign for change (Revenson and Cassell 1991, Watts 1997, McNeill 1999). In contrast, Cancer Black Care, founded in 1995 by a man whose brother had died from cancer, was one of the few groups representing ethnic minority health in our study. At the time of the interview, the group was small and not well networked with other groups.

Within the arthritis area a number of groups have recently been formed by people with relatively rare conditions. An account given by the founder member of one such group illustrates well the process of recognition, attribution and action that leads to group formation. She said that she had met someone else with the same symptoms in an outpatients department and that: 'just finding somebody who understood and didn't think I was going round the bend, it was so helpful'. They decided to form a group and for the first year ran it themselves with the help of their husbands. Litigation initiated by a parallel group against a drug company that had supplied a drug associated with the illness triggered a huge demand for information. She said: '. . . we were absolutely swamped. We had to get more and more people involved and [set up] a committee' (group interview 15). In the case of rare conditions such as this, group members become experts. Specialist scientific knowledge is acquired by various means and combined with lay knowledge. A common aim is to raise awareness about the disease among health professionals and in particular to improve diagnosis at the primary care level.

By contrast, the De Montfort study identified few high profile groups, formed by patients or carers, in the heart and circulatory disease area. Even the British Cardiac Patients Association, set up in 1982, was instigated by doctors working at a specialist hospital undertaking complex heart surgery.

In a study of five US cities, Davidson, Peenebaker and Dickerson (2000) also found that heart groups did not appear among the leading patient support groups. Heart and circulatory disease does not appear to arouse feeling of anger and resentment, or pose a threat to identity, in the same way as the conditions mentioned previously. This may relate to the high incidence of heart disease, the age and sex of those affected, the known links between lifestyle and the disease, and to the forms of clinical intervention available.

We identified some smaller heart groups set up by patients or carers. Cardiac Risk in the Young (1995) was established by a parent whose son was diagnosed with a potentially fatal heart condition, and the Cardiomyopathy Association (1990) was formed by a patient diagnosed with hypertrophic cardiomyopathy, a heart condition associated with Sudden Death Syndrome. Different Strokes, set up in 1996, is a group run by 'younger stroke survivors who recognised and had experienced the then woeful lack of support and shortage of relevant information' (Different Strokes 2003). These conditions are all relatively rare and/or they concern younger people. This may explain the emotional and structural factors driving group formation.

New social movements, some theorists suggest, tend to attract activists from an educated middle class concerned with cultural change, and this is supported by the findings (Gouldner 1979, Rootes 1995). A professional background and previous activism, as well as negative experiences related to the diagnosis and treatment of a disease, were common characteristics of those group organisers. Age may also be an important variable. A number of the groups in our study had been formed by younger people. Some interviewees referred to pressure from younger members to put certain issues – such as genetic testing – on the organisational agenda. The two groups representing older people also referred to grass-roots activism and the importance of 'grey power'.

From the example of heart disease, it is clear that people do not mobilise around all conditions in the same way. Small and Rhodes (2000) note in their study of Cystic Fibrosis, Motor Neurone Disease and Multiple Sclerosis support groups that some members did not attend meetings because they were too ill or because they did not want to associate with people who were at an advanced stage of the illness. More investigation is needed to explore why the barriers to membership and group formation may be greater for some conditions than others.

Shared norms and values: towards a health consumer movement
On the basis of the interview analysis, the De Montfort data indicated that not only was there a common discourse and perceptions within health consumer groups in the same condition area, but that there were also shared values and norms across condition areas providing evidence for a wider health consumer movement. A common discourse has developed, the notion, for example, of a 'cancer journey'; 'living with' an illness, rather than 'suffering from' a disease. The concept of 'a long-term condition' as a broader unifying concept

has tended to replace the more limited and more clinically-oriented 'chronic illness'; the experience of 'carers' as well as 'patients' is considered important, and the notion of the 'expert patient' has developed. As Bourdieu (1991) has suggested, communities are defined by language and perception.

People who speak for groups gain their authority and legitimacy from drawing on the lay experience of living with, or living through, an illness, pain, or loss. This culture has also come to pervade groups whose origins lie in the philanthropic or advocacy tradition. The groups in our data set that were not member groups had appointed people with an illness to their decision-making bodies; had employed them on projects; and had consulted widely with the constituency. All groups in the data set acknowledged that the lay experience brought a particular expertise which added to their claim to speak for patients, whether a group was run by paid officials, or by those with direct experience.

In relation to HIV/AIDS, Epstein (1996) shows that expertise has many facets. It develops from how lay people use scientific, clinical knowledge as well as the lay experience itself. In interviews people spoke of their own struggle to develop knowledge and expertise through consulting specialist professionals, websites and evidence from randomised controlled trials, so that, as one interviewee put it, they knew 'enough to become a doctor'. As Brown (1992: 269) has commented: 'lay persons gather scientific data and other information and also direct and marshall the knowledge and resources of experts in order to understand the epidemiology of the disease'. The Cochrane Collaboration's web-based databases provide global access to research data, and groups in our sample reported using many of these sources as well as getting information directly from experts.

Sharing the subjective experience of living with illness, pain or loss is one aspect of health consumer group activity, but groups may also codify knowledge systematically by collating information and undertaking research. Lay knowledge, like scientific knowledge, is negotiable. It helps both to construct individual and collective identity and contributes to political resources. As most (80%) health consumer groups in the De Montfort study ran helplines and produced pamphlets for the general public (87%), they regarded themselves, and were regarded by other stakeholders interviewed, as repositories of expertise. Many groups analysed helplines to spot emerging trends and to legitimate knowledge claims.

Those interviewed in the De Montfort study also placed a high value on consultative and participatory practices. For membership groups, this ensured cohesion and gave authority to leaders as 'holders' of interests. Schmitter (2001) has used the term 'participatory governance' to refer to new forms of governance that require the engagement of a range of nominally equal interests in decision making. Health consumer groups used a variety of means to communicate with and to involve the membership. Newsletters, special projects, meetings, a branch structure, conferences, fun days, lobbying events and, less frequently, internet chat rooms were used to develop connections between members and the group headquarters.

There was a recognition by virtually all those interviewed that their role was to reflect the concerns of the membership and that interaction was a two-way process. A very small minority of interviewees referred to internal conflicts. Sometimes, a splinter group formed, or a resource or management failure led to a crisis for a group – a reminder that for membership groups, survival depended on their own efforts. Group leaders drew on the expertise of members, both as a matter of principle, and to maintain cohesion. Members looked to the leadership to inform them of policy developments, to manage external relations and to develop a programme of action.

Health consumer groups and the media
Another trend identified in the research was the importance placed by groups on favourable media coverage, and most groups in the data set had appointed policy or media officers, sometimes as a top priority. The accounts given above indicate that media coverage is often crucial to group formation, as it allows others with similar problems or views to be identified. A number of founder members talked of being overwhelmed following media coverage. As Jennings (1999) points out, the media have a strong interest in illness, especially since pain and loss issues reflect both public interest and commercial considerations. The experiences of individuals provide stories, and some groups had a database of members who were willing to tell their story. Data can be filed by region, gender, age and diagnosis and used to select copy for local or national journalists. The British media have tended to be supportive of health consumer groups, perhaps because their main target for criticism has been the medical profession, scientific experts and government.

Not all causes, however, receive equal, or necessarily positive, coverage – hence the importance to health consumer groups of cultivating media contacts. Interviewees from both arthritis and mental health groups complained about being ignored or the subject of adverse coverage. In particular, mental illness was still considered to carry a stigma and groups felt that the tabloid press reinforced negative stereotypes. This view is supported in research by Philo (1996) who found that the reporting of dangerous and psychotic behaviour outweighed the coverage of chronic mental health problems.

Women's health issues receive considerable attention, especially in the broadsheets and in television documentaries. Cancer, and particularly breast cancer, attracts wider coverage than might be expected, in terms of mortality (Henderson and Kitzinger 1999, Saywell, Beattie and Henderson 2000). Some health consumer groups found that media attention could be counterproductive when it diverted attention from the issues that they wished to promote. For example, one breast cancer group said they were trying to get breast cancer for older women on the agenda but had been asked for a story about a young, preferably blonde, mother with a diagnosis of breast cancer. Similarly, some maternity and childbirth groups believed their efforts to reduce technological intervention were undermined by journalists who mocked their 'earth mother' image, and by press reports about celebrities who opted for elective caesareans.

Networking, informal and formal alliances
The De Montfort study identified extensive networking and both informal and formal policy alliances between health consumer groups. There was extensive networking between health consumer groups themselves and between health consumer groups and national consumer organisations such as the Consumers' Association and the National Consumer Council. These extensive inter-connections demonstrate a discourse, a shared assumptive world, and a community of interest between groups, and they support the argument that a clearly defined health consumer movement exists.

In reconstructing their past, a number of interviewees referred to particular defining periods or events that had sparked active networking. In the late-1980s, an informal alliance between carers' groups was established to seek legislative changes to assess carers' needs, and this eventually led to additional payments for carers (Baggott, Allsop and Jones 2004). At around the same time, following intensive lobbying by a range of interconnected groups in the health sector, an opportunity presented itself to shape the maternity service. This led to a new policy on childbirth, endorsed by the Department of Health (DOH 1993).

From the late-1980s, health consumer groups across the board were concerned with the Conservative government's health reforms. These introduced quasi-market principles into the health service and groups feared the consequences. From their own accounts, an informal alliance of patients' groups, the Patients Forum, began meeting around 1990, and was formalised in 1996 as an association of health consumer groups and affiliated professional associations. Concurrently, another alliance of groups with a common interest in chronic illness began to meet. Known as the Long-term Medical Conditions Alliance (LMCA), this group appointed its first paid officer in 1996. Most recently the Mental Health Alliance, a coalition of health consumer groups and professionals opposed to the reform of the 1983 Mental Health Act, forced the Government to withdraw its bill from the 2003 legislative programme. The reforms would have restricted the rights of people with a mental illness receiving care in the community.

Formal alliances are a relatively new phenomenon: 11 were identified in the research. These are made up of clusters of health consumer groups who identify a common interest. Some alliances are large. In April 2003, the LMCA included 112 groups and the Patients Forum had a membership of 81 groups. The consensus among those interviewed was that joining an alliance served a number of purposes. First, it provided an opportunity for learning about how to influence the policy process; second, it improved access to policy networks. Resources could also be shared. Larger and better-established groups supported those less fortunate by providing training and co-ordinating lobbying activity. Groups that joined an alliance had evidently weighed the costs and benefits in terms of their own place in the 'market'. Indeed, a small minority of groups said they saw no advantage in joining an alliance.

In summary, the trends outlined above indicate a health consumer sector that is capable of collective action. It can be argued that the increase in the number of groups formed by people with direct experience of a particular illness has assisted groups across the sector both to construct and defend a situated lay knowledge and to follow participative and consultative practices. These factors have been important in building the trust necessary for collaboration and collective action both within, and across, groups. UK health consumer groups have taken joint action and, from time to time, campaigned effectively to amend or delay legislation (Allsop, Baggott and Jones 2002).

Pain, loss and the formation of protest groups

During the De Montfort study, it became apparent that a few groups in the data set had extended their activities from support and influencing policy to include protest against a 'perceived injurious experience' linked to a claim for redress. In his discussion of pain and loss, Jennings (1999) acknowledges that a range of events associated with illness and other events can impinge sufficiently to cause a threat to identity. Such events may be felt directly, or indirectly when they affect close others such as kin, lovers and carers, but whether action is taken, and in what form, depends on how events are perceived and how responsibility and blame are allocated. In making his argument, Jennings draws implicitly on attribution theory. This was used to explain pathways to disputing by Felstiner, Abel and Sarat (1981) who described the process as 'naming, blaming and claiming'. First, something has to be perceived as injurious; second, someone or something must be blamed; and third, a course of action must be determined.

Felstiner, Abel and Sarat (1981) demonstrated that pathways to dispute arenas are socially-patterned and that they are influenced by a range of social and structural variables. Although they did not investigate group formation and action, their theory is important in understanding the formation of health consumer and particularly, protest groups. In the research, we used the term 'protest group' to categorise groups where the *primary* task was to seek redress where the cause of the injury was attributed to an individual or agency.

A data set of 26 protest groups was identified from those giving written and/or oral evidence to five recent public inquiries (DOH 1994, Health Select Committee 1999, The Bristol Inquiry 2001[5], Royal Liverpool Children's Inquiry 2001, Shipman Inquiry 2002)[6]. Data on these organisations was collected from their websites and from the LexisNexis database, a newspaper archive. The aim was to establish the similarities and differences between protest groups and the more policy-oriented health consumer groups.

Table 2 *Protest groups in the UK in 2003 by date of formation*

Date of formation	Percentage of Groups	Number of Groups
pre-1980	15	4
1981–1990	27	7
1991–to date	58	15
Total	100	26

Source: Protest Group study data set 2003

The data were entered on to a matrix to record selected characteristics such as the date of formation, why a group was established, who was held responsible and blamed for the injurious experience, and the form of redress sought. Table 2 shows a sharp increase in the numbers of groups. Seven groups were established between 1981 and 1990 and 15 were formed in 1991 or after. Groups formed in the 1980s were more likely to be either advocacy and advice groups, such as the Association for the Victims of Medical Accidents (AVMA), the Prevention of Professional Abuse Network (POPAN) and Inquest; or membership groups concerned with people who perceived themselves as damaged by vaccines or medication such as the Vaccine Victims Support Group UK and Battle Against Tranquillisers. Some of these groups had engaged in legal 'class actions' for compensation (Gabe, Gustaffsson and Bury 1991).

The fact that more than half the groups were formed in 1991 or after suggests that numbers have increased. As the total number of groups formed in each period is not known this may be an artefact of the data. Many of the groups referred to themselves as 'victims', a term that Borkman (1999) suggests is a characteristic of 'fledgling' groups. But, the implication is that responsibility for the harm caused lies with another human agent who is blame-worthy. The two largest categories of groups were 1) those formed by people who believed that they were the victim of a medical error or 'adverse event' and 2) groups where members attributed their illness or disability to medicines or vaccines. Anger about a lack of informed consent and the absence of information was a common concern.

A particular feature of group formation was that in many cases there was a geographical clustering of cases and, typically, a particular doctor, nurse or hospital unit was held responsible. Thus, there was a cluster of deaths of children undergoing cardiac surgery in Bristol that led to the formation of the Bristol Heart Children's Action Group. The Rodney Ledward Victim's Support Group and the Action and Support Group for Medical Victims of Richard Neale were formed by women with failed gynaecological operations in Kent and North Yorkshire respectively. A cluster of parents, who found that body parts of their dead children had been retained without consent by the Royal Liverpool children's hospital, (Alder Hey), formed Parents who have Interred their Children Twice (PITY II). Another example was the Tameside Families Support Group formed by people in Hyde, Greater Manchester, who believed that their relatives had been murdered by the infamous general practitioner, the late Harold Shipman.

The people who consider themselves as victims of a particular drug or medicine, as opposed to a particular practitioner or service provider, are usually more widely dispersed. This may make group formation less likely, unless there is a pre-existing group that can identify a trend among its members. For example, the Haemophilia Society, primarily a support group, now campaigns for compensation for people with haemophilia who have been infected with HIV/AIDS and other diseases through blood transfusions.

When people gave evidence to public enquiries, feelings of grief, distress, isolation and anger were commonly cited. If someone speaks out, and this has a resonance with others, a group can form quite rapidly. This is illustrated in written evidence to the House of Commons Health Select Committee inquiry into adverse clinical incidents (Health Select Committee 1999). The founder member of one victim support group described the inaugural meeting attended by 22 women thus:

> Some were far too ill to come to the meeting, yet assured us by telephone of their unconditional support for our group and its objectives . . . most, if not all, of these women did not take legal action, nor did they make a complaint to the hospital where they were treated, since they were (a) too ill and (b) felt they were 'the only one'. They each felt they would simply be one voice 'crying in the wilderness' . . . all of these women have indicated they feel heartened and encouraged by the existence of our Action and Support Group and each is willing and anxious to come forward and tell her story (Written Evidence to the Committee ACI217B).

The quotation underlines the importance of a shared identity but indicates the presence of social entrepreneurs with leadership capability. Although the process of formation of protest groups could not be investigated in detail, it is likely that gossip networks and contact with 'knowledgeables' and coverage of an issue by the local or national media, as with the health consumer groups described above, can play an important role (Allsop and Mulcahy 2001).

Protest groups, however, were more likely to view medical practices as paternalistic and oppressive and to see health professionals as people who withheld information and close ranks against patients when questioned. Protest groups were also highly cynical about the motives of pharmaceutical companies, which they perceived as concerned with profit and not with the long-term effects of their products on patients. In contrast, the health consumer groups in the De Montfort study varied in their attitudes. Many had formed collaborative and productive relationships with professionals and some took funding from pharmaceutical companies, generally for limited and specific purposes.

In terms of size, protest groups tend to be smaller and less long-lived than health consumer groups. If redress is obtained, or indeed if an action fails, they may cease to exist. Some may develop into more broadly-based groups, as has been the case in the mental health sector. It is not known if there is networking and learning between protest groups, although this is suggested by the shared discourse, perceptions and forms of action. Moreover, expert advocacy groups such as the Association for the Victims of Medical Accidents provide advice and are closely networked with the mainstream health consumer movement.

Health consumer groups and the policy process

In the introduction, it was argued that groups have mobilised in response to illness, pain and loss, across a number of different countries. Indeed, many interviewees in the De Montfort study referred to international conferences and contacts. However, political culture and national institutions shape the actions and activities undertaken by health consumer groups. In the UK, health consumer groups tend to use conventional political channels. They aim to raise public awareness of issues, and seek publicity through the media. They often work with professionals and professional associations, and through the political process in Westminster and in Whitehall[7]. The questionnaire data from the De Montfort study showed that contact between health consumer groups and policy makers had increased in frequency in the last three years. Interview data showed extensive contact with civil servants and ministers at various stages in the policy process.

It can be argued that the centralisation of British political institutions – its national, tax-based health service, and a centrally-regulated charity sector – have encouraged the use of conventional channels. In putting pressure on politicians, health consumer groups have pushed on an open door. Both Conservative and Labour administrations have favoured a style of governance that seeks to engage with a range of interests through initiating a range of new participatory practices (Newman 2001 and Daly 2003). In relation to health consumer groups, the De Montfort study showed that civil servants and politicians acknowledged the importance of lay knowledge and expertise in making a contribution to policy development and resource allocation. They have incorporated group representatives in informal networks, on policy development committees, and as members of decision-making bodies. For example, health consumer group representatives were included on committees that drew up the national policy frameworks that established treatment models and standards for a number of conditions such as coronary heart disease and cancer. They are also represented on committees of the National Institute for Clinical Excellence (NICE), a body which examines and recommends cost-effective health technologies for use in the NHS.

There have also been changes in governments' response to protest groups. First, there are now alternative pathways for dispute resolution for those who perceive themselves as harmed by health professionals (Mulcahy *et al.* 1999). Second, where groups form and it is accepted that there is wrong-doing, the establishment of an inquiry is a favoured strategy. The aim is to gather information, to provide an audience for those who have suffered, and to learn the lessons for policy. There is a discourse of partnership and resolution. Some of the terminology has been influenced by health consumer groups. For example, the term 'expert patient' (also used in US initiatives) has been adopted in plans for services for people with a long-term illness (DOH 2001) and a recent consultation document on clinical negligence, which proposes strategies to provide care and support for victims, is termed *Making Amends* (DOH 2003). Professional bodies, and even pharmaceutical companies, in pursuit of their own interests, also include patients' groups and consumers directly in discussions on policy proposals to add legitimacy to their activities.

Conclusion

This chapter argues that a broadly-based health consumer movement has developed over the past decade, and it has been based largely on a belief in the validity of lay experience. Health consumer groups have a situated knowledge which draws on personal experience, but incorporates other forms of expertise. The people who represent groups may themselves speak from personal experience but they also legitimate their position through drawing on the experience of their members and this is achieved by operating consultative and participatory practices. Health consumer groups themselves develop both loose networks of connection and more structured alliances, and these are mirrored in policy-level networks. Protest groups can be considered as an important sub-set of health consumer groups, where the attribution of responsibility and blame is more sharply focused on an individual or agency and where there is an emphasis on redress rather than on service change. It is probable that the community of interest between groups has been encouraged by being drawn into the national policy arena and by developing closer links with other interests in health care. Arguably, these changes indicate a health consumer movement.

This, however, says little about the powers of health consumer groups either individually or collectively. It may simply be that inclusion in the policy process leads to incorporation. That is, health consumer groups could simply become actors in a process that provides enhanced legitimacy to governments as they pursue their own larger agenda. It is useful to bring in health consumer groups to curb the monopoly powers of health professionals and to build public support for particular health policies. Apart from seeking alliances with more powerful interests, health consumer groups, whether acting individually or in combination, have few power resources except possibly through the mobilisation of media support.

It could also be argued that the health consumer movement is actually a collection of disparate interests and that involvement in the policy process will exacerbate differences. There are certainly tensions. Health consumer group resources are limited, and time spent on government committees is time not spent on member activities. Some groups and condition areas are closer to policy makers than others. There are insiders and outsiders; some issues are on the agenda and others are not. Leaders may find themselves separated from grass-roots activists with other agendas. Political opportunities for participation may cease to be on offer. Nevertheless, despite these caveats, health care politics have been significantly changed by the presence of a new set of actors within the health policy process.

Acknowledgements

The De Montfort study was funded by the Economic and Social Research Council Grant Number R000237888. We would also like to thank the people who reviewed the earlier draft of the chapter for their comments.

Notes

1 There was a small overlap (2 groups) between the De Montfort study and the Protest Group study.
2 Inclusion and exclusion criteria were used in both the De Montfort study and the Protest Group study.
3 Each organisation was telephoned before the questionnaire was sent out, and the person answering the telephone asked to identify the member of staff who was in charge of policy activity.
4 Examples of condition-based groups included larger groups such as MIND (National Association of Mental Health) and the Stroke Association, but also smaller groups such as Cancer Black Care and Action on Pre-Eclampsia. Examples of the population-based groups included Help the Aged and Action for Sick Children and of formal alliances, the Genetic Interest Group and the Long-term Medical Conditions Alliance.
5 Bristol Inquiry: groups that took part in a seminar on patient empowerment undertaken as part of the inquiry were included in the sample.
6 Groups that gave evidence to phase one of the inquiry, the report of the second phase has yet to be published.
7 Westminster – refers to Parliament (House of Commons/House of Lords), Whitehall – refers to government departments and central executive institutions such as the Prime Minister's Office.

References

Allsop, J., Baggott, R. and Jones, K. (2002) Health consumer groups and the policy process. In Henderson, S. and Peterson, A. *Consuming Health: the Commodification of Health Care.* London and New York: Routledge.

Allsop, J. and Mulcahy, L. (2001) Dealing with clinical complaints. In Vincent, C. (ed.) *Clinical Risk Management: Enhancing Patient Safety.* 2nd Edition. London: BMA Books.

Baggott, R., Allsop, J. and Jones, K. (2004 forthcoming) *Speaking for Patients and Carers: Health Consumer Groups and the Policy Process.* Basingstoke: Palgrave.

Bastian, H. (1998) Speaking up for ourselves, *International Journal of Technological Assessment in Health Care,* 14, 1, 3–23.

Berridge, V. (2002) AIDS and the rise of the patient? Activist organisation and HIV/AIDS in the UK in the 1980s and 1990s, *Medizin, Gesellschaft und Geschichte,* 21, 109–24.

Borkman, T. (1999) *Understanding Self-Help/Mutual Aid: Experiential Learning in the Commons.* New Brunswick, New Jersey: Rutgers University Press.

Brown, P. (1984) Marxism, social psychology, and the sociology of mental health, *International Journal of Health Services,* 14, 2, 237–408.

Brown, P. (1992) Popular epidemiology and toxic waste contamination: lay and professional ways of knowing, *Journal of Health and Social Behaviour,* 33, 267–81.

Brown, P., Mayer, B., Zavestovski, S., Luebke, T., Mandelbaum, J. and Mc Cormick, S. (2003) The health politics of asthma: environmental justice and collective illness experience in the United States, *Social Science and Medicine,* 57, 453–64.

Bourdieu, P. (1991) *Language and Symbolic Power.* Cambridge: Policy Press.

Bury, M. (1982) Chronic illness as a biographical description, *Sociology of Health and Illness,* 4, 167–82.

Byrne, P. (1997) *Social Movements in Britain.* London: Routledge.

Campbell, J. and Oliver, M. (1996) *Disability Politics.* London: Routledge.

Charmaz, K. (1983) Loss of self: a fundamental form in suffering in the chronically ill, *Sociology of Health and Illness,* 5, 168–98.

Clement-Jones, V. (1985) Cancer and beyond: the formation of BACUP, *British Medical Journal,* 291, 1021–3.

Crossley, N. (1999) Fish, field, habitus and madness: the first wave mental health users movement in Great Britain, *British Journal of Sociology,* 50, 4, 647–70.

Daly, M. (2003) Governance and social policy, *Journal of Social Policy,* 32, 1, 113–28.

Davidson, K.P., Pennebaker, J.W. and Dickerson, S.S. (2000) Who talks? The social psychology of illness support groups, *American Psychologist,* 55, 2, 205–17.

Department of Health (1993) *Changing Childbirth, Report of the Expert Materity Group.* Chair, Baroness Cumberledge. London: HMSO.

Department of Health (1994) *Being Heard: a Review Committee on NHS Complaints Procedures.* Chair (now Sir), Alan Wilson. Leeds: Department of Health.

Department of Health (2001) *The Expert Patient a New Approach to Disease Management for the 21st Century.* London: Department of Health.

Department of Health (2003) *Making Amends: a Consultation Paper Setting Out Proposals for Reforming the Approach to Clinical Negligence in the NHS.* London: Department of Health.

Different Strokes (2003) Introduction [www] Available from: http://www.differentstrokes.co.uk/intro/htm (Accessed 20 June 2003).

Doyal, L. (ed.) (1998) *Women and Health Services.* Buckingham: Open University Press.

Epstein, S. (1996) *Impure Science: Aids, Activism, and the Politics of Knowledge.* Berkley and Los Angeles, California: University of California Press.

Felstiner, W., Abel, R. and Sarat, A. (1981) The emergence and transformation of disputes: naming, blaming, claiming . . . , *Law and Society Review,* 15, 631–54.

Gabe, J., Gustafsson, U. and Bury, M. (1991) Mediating illness – newspaper coverage of tranquilliser dependence, *Sociology of Health and Illness*, 13, 332–53.

Giddens, A. (1979) *Central Problems of Social Theory*. London: Macmillan.

Gouldner, A.W. (1979) *The Future of Intellectuals and the Rise of the New Class*. New York: Oxford University Press.

Habermas, J. (1984) *The Theory of Collective Action: Volume 1: Reason and Rationalisation of Society*. Boston, Mass: Beacon Press.

Health Select Committee House of Commons (1999) *Procedures Related to Adverse Clinical Incidents and Outcomes in Medical Care*. London: The Stationery Office.

Henderson, L. and Kitzinger, J. (1999) The human drama of genes: media representations of inherited breast cancer, *Sociology of Health and Illness*, 21, 560–78.

Jennings, M.K. (1999) Political responses to pain and loss: presidential address at the 1998 American Political Science Association, *American Political Science Review*, 93, 1, 1–15.

Levy, L. (1981) The National Schizophrenia Fellowship: a British self-help group, *Social Psychiatry*, 16, 129–35.

Lewin, E. and Olesen, V. (1985) *Women, Health and Healing: Towards a New Perspective*. London: Tavistock Publications.

McNeill, J. (1999) Cancerlink: helping people help themselves, *European Journal of Cancer Care*, 8, 1, 12–15.

Martin, G. (2001) Social movements welfare and social policy: a critical analysis, *Critical Social Policy*, 21, 3, 361–83.

Melucci, A. (1989) *Nomads of the Present: Social Movements and Individual Needs in Contemporary Society*. Philadelphia: Temple University Press.

Meyer, D.S. and Whittier, N. (1994) Social movement spillover, *Social Problems*, 41, 2, 277–98.

Mulcahy, L., Selwood, M., Summerfield, L. and Netten, A. (1999) *Mediating Medical Negligence Claims an Option for the Future?* London: The Stationery Office.

Newman, J. (2001) *Modernising Governance: New Labour, Policy and Society*. London: Sage.

Philo, G. (ed.) (1996) *Media and Mental Distress*. London: Longman.

Revenson, T.A. and Cassell, J.B. (1991) An exploration of leadership in a medical mutual help organisation, *American Journal of Psychology*, 19, 5, 683–97.

Rogers, A. and Pilgrim, D. (1991) Pulling down churches: accounting for the British Mental Health Users Movement, *Sociological of Health and Illness*, 13, 2, 129–48.

Rogers, A. and Pilgrim, D. (2001) *Mental Health Policy in Britain*. Basingstoke: Palgrave.

Rootes, C. (1995) The new class: the higher educated and the new politics. In Maheu, L. (ed.) *Social Movements and Social Classes*. London: Sage.

Royal Liverpool Children's Inquiry (2001) *Royal Liverpool Children's Inquiry Report*. Chair, Michael Redfern QC. London: The Stationery Office.

Saywell, C., Beattie, L. and Henderson, L. (2000) Sexualised illness: the newsworthy body in media representations of breast cancer. In Potts, L. (ed.) *Ideologies of Breast Cancer: Feminist Perspectives*. London: Macmillan.

Schmitter, P. (2001) Participatory governance in a multi-level context. In Grote, J.R. and Gbikpi, B. (eds) *Participatory Governance: Political and Societal Implications*. Opladen: Leske and Budrick.

Shipman Inquiry (2002) *Independent Public Inquiry into the Issues Arising from the Case of Harold Frederick Shipman*. Chair, Dame Janet Smith. London: The Stationery Office.

Simon, B. and Klandermans, B. (2001) Politicized collective identity: a social psychological analysis, *American Psychologist*, 56, 4, 319–31.

Small, M. and Rhodes, P. (2000) *Too Ill to Talk? User Involvement and Palliative Care*. London: Routledge.

Tew, M. (1998) *Safer Childbirth? A Critical History of Maternity Care*. 3rd Edition. London: Free Association.

The Bristol Inquiry (2001) *Learning from Bristol, Public Inquiry into Children's Heart Surgery at the Bristol Royal Infirmary 1984–1995*. Chair, Professor (now Sir), Ian Kennedy. London: The Stationery Office.

Watts, E.J. (1997) Cancer self-help groups are underused, *British Medical Journal*, 315, 812.

Weeks, J., Aggleton, P., McKevitt, C., Parkinson, K. and Taylor-Labourn, A. (1996) Community and contracts: tensions and dilemmas in the voluntary sector response to HIV and AIDS, *Policy Studies*, 17, 2, 107–23.

Weeks, J., Holland, J. and Waites, M. (2003) *Sexualities and Society*. Cambridge: Policy Press.

Williams, G. (1984) The genesis of chronic illness, *Sociology of Health and Illness*, 6, 175–200.

Wood, B. (2000) *Patient Power? The Politics of Patients Associations in Britain and America*. Buckinghamshire: Open University Press.

Chapter 5

Regenerating movements: embryonic stem cells and the politics of potentiality
Chris Ganchoff

Introduction

Human embryonic stem cell (ESC) technologies are being heralded by many, both inside and outside biomedical institutions, as revolutionary break-throughs for the amelioration of a variety of pathologies. While stem cell-based therapeutics are still in an early phase of development, their creation from ESC precursors has provoked tremendous controversies across the social landscape. By the mid-1990s, the epistemological and material conditions were fertile for the discovery and articulation of the human embryonic stem cell and the development of what is now referred to as 'regenerative medicine' (Aldhous 2001, Dominguez-Bendala *et al.* 2002, Strom *et al.* 2002). In November 1998, researchers at the University of Wisconsin led by James Thomson published a report in *Science* that has become a focal point in the recent history of ESCs. The Wisconsin team ended the report by detailing the potential benefits of basic research understandings of ESC developmental dynamics, and by listing the potential therapeutic interventions that could be produced (Thomson *et al.* 1998: 1146–7). Thomson and his colleagues downplayed the allusion to ethical difficulties involved in their research, limiting comment to one statement about the 'ethical and practical reasons' for conducting human and non-human primate ESC experimenta-tion (1998: 1145). Instead, the Wisconsin team highlighted the benefits that could be gained, such as preventing infertility, birth defects, Parkinson's disease and diabetes mellitus, as well as promoting advances in cell trans-plantation and preventing immune rejection (1998: 1146–7).

From this post-1998-charged social environment, regenerative medicine and ESC research have become embroiled in widening political debates (Bonnicksen 2002, Holland *et al.* 2001). Recently, ESC technology has been linked to possible breakthroughs in a variety of illnesses and conditions (Daley 2002, MacKay 2000, Snyder and Vescovi 2000, Stanworth and New-land 2001). Resources from both public and private sources have begun flowing towards these domains, and especially in the cases of diabetes and Parkinson's disease, significant 'bandwagons' (Fujimura 1996) have gained momentum, pushing for ESC-based cures for these diseases. These bandwagons include bench scientists, clinical researchers, patients and their families, disease-specific advocates and activists, biomedical technicians of various stripes, lawyers and legal scholars, government officials and regula-tors, as well as a menagerie of corporate figures from pharmaceutical and biotechnology industries, who often span and inhabit many of the aforementioned groups.

For this chapter, the focus is on a subset of the actors implicated in debates over ESC research, chosen because their 'work activities' produce perspectives that articulate various connections (Clarke 1990: 20). This method comes out of the social worlds tradition in sociological research (Becker 1982, Clarke and Gerson 1990, Fujimura 1988, Strauss 1978 are a few examples). Clarke, for example, argues that there are three major types of social worlds: production worlds; communal worlds; and social movements. However, she goes on to state that 'mixed worlds are both possible and common' (Clarke 1990: 19). The groups in each world, though they may dimly recognise each other, are committed to lines of action whose intersections produce intriguing and difficult questions and problems.

In this chapter I argue for analysing social movements as operating within a *field of biotechnology*. Coming through the social movement traditions, as well as science and technology studies, this article will compare understandings of ESC technologies in four different social movements while foregrounding the concept of the field.

Social movements and fields of struggles

Much of extant social movement theory explains collective action through recourse to strategy; this is apparent in the emphasis on the cognitive and signifying processes that underlie the framing perspective (Benford 1997, Snow and Benford 1992, Snow *et al.* 1986), as well as the attention paid to organisational politics and structural opportunities by the resource mobilisation and contentious politics approaches (Jenkins 1983, McAdam 1999, McAdam *et al.* 2001, McCarthy and Zald 1977, Tarrow 1998). Without a doubt, seeing social movement actors as rational and reflective is critical for understanding the importance of social movements in liberal democracies.

Political process theory has been challenged on its supposed 'structural bias' (Goodwin and Jasper 1999: see the special issue of *Sociological Forum* for the complete debate), and I will not rehash those arguments here (Swidler 1986, Taylor and Whittier 1995). By now, cultural, symbolic and corporeal processes have all been explored within the purview of social movement scholarship (Goodwin *et al.* 2001, Guidry *et al.* 2000, Jasper 1997, Johnston and Klandermans 1995, Klandermans and Johnston 1995, Klawiter 1999, Kroll-Smith and Floyd 1997, Taylor and Whittier 1995). This body of work shows that practices of signification and embodiment are not just supplements to strategic thought and action, but rather that culture and structure are deeply intertwined.

One way to access the clumsy binary of culture/structure is by focusing on *fields* in which social movement activity occurs. Fields have been important for various strands of social theory. For example, Pierre Bourdieu has knitted together dispositions (habitus), different forms of capital, and the arenas of conflict that are both constitutive of social identities as well as domains of conflict over expertise and representation (fields) into a theoretical architecture that takes on distinctions of culture and structure (Bourdieu 1990, Bourdieu and Wacquant 1992). While Bourdieu does talk specifically about the field of science and scientific reason, it is always in terms of *scientists* and their relationships to the scientific field (Bourdieu 1975, 1991). In other words, the field is composed of, and regulated by, experts who have specific dispositions towards the objective and potential structures of the scientific field, including scientific capital. Scientific reason thus takes form through the conflicts between strategies of monopolisation of the field by the dispositions of those enmeshed within it. For Bourdieu, fields are generative sites from the inside out; to enter, one has to accept certain presuppositions (the 'doxa'), and then begin the struggle to accumulate forms of capital. This set of processes extends the contiguous field, and pushes its 'autonomisation' from other fields.

Bourdieu's conceptualisation of the field is certainly important. It does however have limitations; namely, it does not account for the ways in which fields are susceptible to the influence of a wide variety of actors. One way to address this missing aspect is to conceptualise fields as essentially open, and crosscut by the movement of objects and actors. For example, Arjun Appadurai describes fields as 'global cultural flows' that are fragmented into multiple terrains (1996: 33). The relationships between these terrains are complex and uneven. In Appadurai's formulation, it is the doxa of a field that have become *disjunctive*; that is, rather than internally unified around a set of shared presuppositions, fields are fragmenting and travelling around the globe by constructing new possibilities for social life (1996). These new sites of sociability fall across the spectrum, from expert to lay, human to non-human, and play a part in constituting the field of biotechnology. This analysis foregrounds the potential for new social relations that are dependent upon the intersections of identity and space.

The field of biotechnology

Two interrelated aspects illustrate the productive nature of the field of biotechnology. The first aspect is the emergence and proliferation of reflexive identities. Phil Brown and colleagues highlight this aspect through their discussion of *embodied health movements* (Brown *et al.* 2004). They argue that embodied health movements (EHMs) are a subset of health social movements, and can be thought of as 'boundary movements', as they exist at the intersections of different institutional and epistemic configurations. The authors pay close attention to the formation of a *politicised collective illness identity* that arises out of both the intersubjective experience of suffering as well as the shared political positions of marginality that come with being diagnosed with a poorly understood or characterised condition. These identities are reflexive in that they are self-fashioned. In other words, while people are subject to biomedical authority, this does not mean they are passive victims. Rather, they build identities through the multiple worlds of biomedicine and social movements.

The production of an imagined space within which various politicised collective illness identities exist is the second aspect of the field of biotechnology. Identities always take shape in relation to some context. One way of schematising this context is through the concept of *biomedicalization* (Clarke *et al.* 2003). Biomedicalisation, which builds on the concept of medicalization (the process of turning social problems into medical phenomena) is the *intensification* of the interpenetration of institutions, organisations, ideologies and bodies under the aegis of health and illness. In other words, it is the 'reorganization' of contemporary biomedicine 'from the inside out' (2003: 2). This means not only the relationships between institutions, actors and technologies, but also the reconsolidation of the very idea of health within an individualized framework of *health maintenance*. That is, health and illness have become the province of constant individual and institutional surveillance, through fitness and dieting plans, as well as genetic testing and new forms of medical imaging. Actors travel through these spaces, albeit to alternate degrees and with different repercussions.

There is a recursivity between biomedical identities and biotechnological spaces; this is what marks the field of biotechnology as generative. As fragments of the body, such as organs, tissues and cells, have become abstracted from this dynamic, they become endowed with potentiality. This potentiality has many forms; it can take shape as the hope for an imagined therapeutic intervention, as well as commercial hype generated by those with investments in biotechnology. This project draws out some of these tensions through a series of interviews, as well as document and website analyses, with actors engaged with the politics of ESC research. These interviews are part of a larger project that is looking at the emergence of embryonic stem cell research, and debates around the ownership of human biological materials. Ten interviews were conducted with actors in various organisations, including a patent law firm, a venture capital organisation, science advocacy movements (Coalition for the Advancement of Medical Research and Research America), patient advocacy groups (Parkinson's Action Network, Michael J. Fox Foundation, and the Juvenile Diabetes Research Foundation), a biotechnology trade organisation (Bay Area Biosciences Center), a professional association (American Society for Cell Biology), and one of the authors of California's 2002 stem cell research legislation.

Patient advocacy groups (PAGs)

The Parkinsons's Action Network (PAN), founded in 1991 in Northern California, works on multiple fronts in the fight against Parkinson's disease (PD), a neurodegenerative condition that results in the death of specific neurons which release a neurotransmitter called dopamine. According to the PAN website (www.parkinsonsaction.org), PD affects 'approximately 1 million Americans, approximately 40 per cent are under the age of 60'. This means that PD affects a relatively small population when compared with other afflictions, such as cancer or heart disease, or even other neurodegenerative diseases like Alzheimer's disease, which strikes 'approximately 4 million Americans' (www.alz.org). However, because of the nature of PD, it has become a major candidate for potential cellular therapies, including ESC-based interventions (Arenas 2002, Borlongan and Sanberg 2002, Brundin and Hagell 2001, Lindvall and Hagell 2001). Thus PD is often mentioned in conjunction with ESC research. PAN, as an organisation, is an enthusiastic supporter of ESC research, and is considered by some as the 'stem cell organisation' (interview 5/8/03).

PAN's work includes supporting legislation at a federal level intended to help cure PD, as well as organising on a grassroots level to increase awareness about PD and potential therapies or cures for PD. PAN's grassroots organising is closely tied to its legislative agenda, as local fieldworkers play a central role in co-ordinating various political functions, such as letter-writing or phone-calling campaigns. Thus, the majority of PAN's work is decentralised, and tailored to the local political environment.

John and Carol (all names are pseudonyms), two PAN activists, both spoke with awe and excitement over the possibilities of ESCs for curing PD. This excitement has been fostered by the potential of ESCs to be coaxed into forming dopamine-producing neurons. But their enthusiasm also has to do with the conjunction of biography, aetiology and politics.

As a neurodegenerative disease, PD is idiopathic; different people are affected in different ways. While PD can ultimately lead to death, there is typically a long period of time from initial onset or diagnosis to death. This affords a window of opportunities, including activism. As Carol pointed out, activism is as much work as her former career, which was truncated by the disease:

It takes away your ability to just move along the path that you've been on. Virtually everyone at some point has to stop working because of it. It's not that you can't work, it's become unreliable. You can't work all the time. You don't know when you'll be able to work, you can't work as fast. You've become unemployable, more than not being able to work. I mean, we work a lot, but it's at all hours of the day and night . . . So it's important to realise that you can 'work'. You can do things, and advocacy is one of the important things you can do because it's so self-fulfilling. So that's why it's an important distinction (Interview, 8 May 2003).

For Carol, taking part in PD activism is part of the process of forming a politicised collective illness identity (Brown et al. 2004). This process leads her not only to meet other activists, but also to understand the significance of ESCs as a potential therapy. Through interaction with others afflicted with PD, Carol and John went through a process of self-redefinition. That is, the self begins to understand itself as *similar to* a group of others, perhaps formerly viewed as foreign. For example, Carol used the metaphor of the leper colony to articulate the connectedness she feels:

> But I think of other communities, like leper colonies. I mean, generally leper colonies, they weren't voluntary by any means, but I'm sure there were consolations of living with each other. Because when we get together with other 'Parkies', inevitably someone will say, 'Oh, God! It is so nice. I don't have to explain myself' (Interview, 8 May 2003).

Feeling at home, not having to explain oneself or one's disposition, creates the conditions for a *proto-citizenship*. Warwick Anderson points out that at Culion, a leper colony in the Philippines, medical authority was enmeshed within a process of citizenship, which for the residents of the colony, directed them 'toward a contained, therapeutic future'. Anderson argues that the leper colony was a 'miniature . . . both bounded yet infinitely expandable' of the colonial control of the Philippines by the USA (Anderson 1998). While Carol's future has more degrees of freedom than those at Culion, for whom full citizenship was always deferred, the domains of health, potentiality and citizenship are brought together within the field of biotechnology. Rather than miniaturising power relations, PAN cultivates the unfolding of the illness experience, and its recoding within the political technologies (Faubion 2000: 403) of social movements.

Science advocacy movements
Science advocacy movements, in the sense used here, have both older and newer forms in the field of biotechnology. By science advocacy movement, I am referring to organised groups and/or coalitions of actors who push for a pro-science agenda. There are organisations, such as the American Association for the Advancement of Science (AAAS) founded in 1848, that attempt to influence federal science policy; the AAAS even weighed in on the stem cell issue (Teich 2002). A pro-science agenda comprises multiple concerns, including increasing government funding for scientific research, relaxing regulatory oversight on scientists or their work, and/or increasing public visibility of scientific endeavours and concerns. Several of these groups are currently active in the United States, one of which is the Coalition for the Advancement of Medical Research (CAMR).

CAMR emerged in 2001 out of the ashes of an earlier coalition known as Patient's Coalition for Urgent Research (Patient's CURe). After Patient's CURe's dissolution, several former members of that coalition formed CAMR, which has taken an active role in lobbying for ESC research as well as therapeutic (as opposed to reproductive) cloning. An activist involved with CAMR, Stephanie, described their organising efforts. She spoke about how CAMR attempts to produce a unified message:

So, as a coalition we were able to get the message out, not to just our membership, but the memberships of everyone involved. So CAMR for instance is developing a set of talking points, that could then be passed along to every CAMR member and CAMR's database of advocates, who we've collected over the years, that could then also be sent out to . . . Christopher Reeve Paralysis Foundation could send it out to their advocacy network, Juvenile Diabetes Research Foundation could send it out to their members, Parkinson's Action Network – so you're getting this consistent voice with a consistent message of why it is that this is important and why it is that we all need to weigh in. So it's extremely complementary to have a coalition advocating on behalf of science, all having the same message and advancing the potential to the best of our abilities (Interview, 23 May 2003).

CAMR's work produces important effects within the field of biotechnology, including amplification of a message through repetition, and ramification of the message into the smallest corners of social life. The first effect has been termed *frame amplification* (Snow *et al.* 1986). This term, developed by Snow and colleagues, encompasses two interrelated elements: value amplification and belief amplification (Snow *et al.* 1986). During the course of recent ESC controversies, the value that CAMR has amplified is the importance of scientific research. This is articulated through the understandings of ESCs versus adult stem cells (ASCs). Some groups opposed to ESC research attempt to drive a wedge between ASCs and ESCs, claiming that ASCs offer better hope for therapeutics, or are morally preferable experimental objects (see below). CAMR, on the other hand, supports ASC and ESC research by seeing both as part of the same continuum:

The reason why you're hearing so much more lately about new discoveries in adult stem cells is because of what we're learning from embryonic stem cells, and they're actually transferring that knowledge . . . We'll actually have more breakthroughs in embryonics by looking at the pre-embryonic state. Well, if you learn how to turn them on and off from a pre-embryonic state, you can apply that to embryonic, you can apply that to umbilical cord, you can apply that to adult – all the advances – the knowledge can be transferred, and it's only going to help everything to move forward faster and smarter by obtaining as much knowledge (Interview, 23 May 2003).

Stephanie locates ESCs within a lineage of cellular life, and emphasises the importance of time for regenerative medicine. This sets up a relation of equivalency between objects of research. Thus, ASCs and ESCs are equally important for biomedical science, and the forfeiture of one ultimately impedes research on the other.

Belief amplification is the second aspect of frame amplification. The belief that follows from the value of unencumbered research is the sense that ESCs represent a new paradigm of medicine:

We think these are the early steps to new treatments. I would say the way that we understand pharmaceuticals today – you know, pharmaceuticals are for the 20th century what cell transplantation will be for the 21st century. It will be a new avenue of medicine. I don't think it will ever be in the way of pharmaceuticals the way we know them now (Interview, 23 May 2003).

Here, Stephanie consolidates the history of ESC research within the scope of medical progress writ large. This belief sets ESCs apart from other forms of treatment, while still locating them within a series. Both the value of unrestricted scientific research and the belief in the transformation of medicine are amplified as they move through the coalitional circuitry. By organising around a single issue, or closely-related issues such as ESCs and cloning, CAMR is able to build a coalition that houses different patient advocacy groups (PAGs), as well as universities and trade organisations.

Larger umbrella movements like CAMR play an important role in structuring the field of biotechnology. While PAGs translate and co-ordinate the idiosyncratic experiences of specific diseases or conditions, groups like CAMR conduct a second order translation; they provisionally unify the diverse worlds of health and illness as a political force within the field. CAMR thus both consolidates and extends the field of biotechnology through the processes of translation and amplification.

Frozen embryo defenders
Since, at the present time, ESCs are derived from human embryos, there are contingents of actors actively opposed to ESC research, as well as groups that remain ambivalent or silent on the matter. Many Christian organisations, such as the Christian Medical Association and the Christian Medical and Dental Associations (CM&DA) oppose ESC research. This discourse often invokes not only the histories of human experimentation, but also the ethics of informed consent. An example of this moral register is from the CM&DA website:

Scientists often seek to push the limits of knowledge, which can result in productive perseverance or horrific ethical compromise. The tragic results of utilitarian human experimentation have been revealed in the Nazi experiments on prisoners at Dachau, the experiments on black syphilis patients at Tuskegee Institute, and the forced hepatitis infection experiments on mentally handicapped children at Willowbrook State School in New York. Good ends do not justify unethical means – including killing human beings. Using already-harvested ES cells would violate longstanding refusals to use evidence derived from unethical human experimentation (www.cmdahome.org).

Compared to CAMR's belief amplification, CM&DA locates ESC research in a different historical trajectory: that of the dystopian side of medical experimentation. This history of medical violence, while the opposite of Stephanie's history of medical progress, contributes to the materialisation of anti-ESC research movements. One movement that has sought to counter the destruction of frozen embryos is Nightlight Christian Adoptions (NCA).

NCA was founded in 1959, and has three adoption divisions: international, domestic and embryo. The embryo adoption programme is called Snowflakes. Snowflakes was formed in 1997, as a result of several events. The first was the rise of *in vitro* fertilization (IVF) as an extremely popular method of assisted reproduction, which has opened up new sets of questions and political positions (Kirejczyk 2000, Mulkay 1997, Valone 1998). Second was a 1996 decision by the Human Fertilization & Embryology Authority of the UK to dispose of 3,300 frozen embryos (Kennedy & Kallenbach 1996). This 'massacre'[1] caused considerable unease among US Catholics, including a couple from Fallbrook, CA, John and Marlene Strege. At that time, the Streges were having trouble conceiving through IVF[2]. Marlene Strege was friends with the executive director of NCA, and in 1997, the two began to talk about the importance of embryo adoption out of the crowded IVF liquid nitrogen holding tanks (Interview, 15 May 2003). Finally, in March 1997, the *Los Angeles Times* reported that there were possibly over 100,000 embryos in storage at IVF clinics in the US (Dobnik 1998). This combination of events led to the formation of Snowflakes.

During the interview with Theresa, who is involved with Snowflakes, she stressed their opposition to reducing frozen embryos to property or commodities, due to a belief that the frozen embryo is the equivalent of a mature person (this is also stated in the embryo adoption agreement). IVF clinics are referred to as 'orphanages'; frozen embryos as 'brothers and sisters'. However, in order to move an embryo out of an IVF clinic for implantation into a woman's womb, two critical functions must be standardised. The first is the construction of a contract between all the partners involved, which operates as a memorandum of understanding. The second is the physical trafficking of the embryo from place to place.

As for the first function, the legal status of embryo adoption is based on regular adoption; there is an 'embryo adoption agreement' similar to an adoption agreement for an infant or child. There are, however, no legal precedents for this kind of adoption, and Snowflakes has modified the agreement to reflect the opinion of the courts that the embryo constitutes a form of property. Therefore, the embryo agreement is recognised in a court of law as a transfer of property, not as an adoption. In terms of the second function, Snowflakes co-ordinates the logistical requirements for movement of an embryo. In the adoption agreement, it states that NCA, 'assumes custody of the embryos transferred', as well as assisting with the 'place-ment of frozen embryos for adoption' (Stoddart 2003: 4–5). Snowflakes contracts out with Federal Express to ship embryos, across state lines if the need arises, but only within the United States[3]. Thus, these two func-tions contribute to the status of the frozen embryo as both *a person* and *a commodity*.

This liminality of the frozen embryo is a critical aspect of the field of biotechnology. The processes involved with 'becoming a thing' or 'becom-ing a person' involve multiple social worlds, including, in this case, assisted reproduction, legal arenas and modes of transportation. While Snowflakes opposes the reduction of frozen embryos to commodities, their work brings the domains of the human and the thing closer together. These domains, rather than being contradictory, are contiguous, perhaps overlapping. The blurred boundary between person and thing, embodied by the frozen embryo, is made intelligible within the field of biotechnology.

Biotechnology advocates
Much like the history of citizen/consumer/patient organising, sectors of indus-try, business and the professions have organised for various, sometimes-conflicting reasons, including professional dominance, regulatory control and/or market dominance. The category of 'biotechnology', while housing different, often contentious boosters and dissenters, has always been closely tied to industrial activity (Bud 1993, Gaudillière and Löwy 1998). In the United States during the 1970s and 1980s, the biotechnology industry bloomed and exploded into one of the most dominant economic sectors (some examples include Brodwin 2000, Heinberg 1999, Krimsky 1991, Rabinow 1996, Sylvester and Klotz 1983, Thackray 1998). One manifestation of this explosion is the Bay Area Biosciences Center, or BayBio.

BayBio was formed in 1990 as a way to promote biotechnological devel-opment in the San Francisco Bay area (www.baybio.org). From a field perspective, BayBio can be thought of as a social movement. As I have argued, potentiality is a central aspect of the field of biotechnology. BayBio offers a vision of this potentiality; this was clearly articulated in a 2003 report from the Office of the Governor of the State of California, with BayBio listed as a participant[4] (Le Merle and Michels 2003). The report identified several 'Key trends and challenges', including 'Growing public interest in the ethics of life sciences' (2003: 11). Recognising that ESC research and regenerative medicine could produce uneasy (or uncontrol-lable) public reactions, the report knits together the economic and the ethical imperatives of biotechnology: 'To ensure the continued success of the region's Life Science cluster, industry, government and the public will need to communicate openly so as to develop a shared vision of what is do-able – and what is right to do' (2003: 11). BayBio plays a major role in the pro-duction of this version of public transparency, which conflates the pragmatic and moral visions of biotechnology. Producing and disseminating this vision of civic biotechnology, much like CAMR does vis-à-vis biomedical research, positions BayBio as a social movement.

While BayBio focuses on organising the biotechnology industry in the Bay Area, it also makes connections with universities and PAGs. Barbara, a former director of BayBio, acknowledged that there is a connection between BayBio and local PAGs in terms of the ways in which ESC research is framed:

> Well, of course, most of them [PAGs] are looking for somebody to circulate out their announcements for their fundraisers, which is a critical thing [laughter] . . . And so we basically play the role of framing the issue on economic terms – jobs generated, how it makes money – if you manage to do research and it eventually spins out into companies and licensing fees for the universities and stuff, and I think it's nice to have some groups that complement each other but don't repeat the same thing (Interview, 20 May 2003).

On the one hand, Barbara jokes about the instrumental aspect of the relationship; like CAMR and orphan disease groups, there are elements of frame amplification and ramification as BayBio and PAGs circulate messages. On the other hand, Barbara reveals that there is a deeper division of framing labour, which takes the form of a tacit agreement. This is a function of the ecology of the field of biotechnology. In other words, there was no formal organisational agreement for PAGs to focus on the corporeal effects of disease and BayBio to focus on the economic end. Nonetheless, the arrangement has been provisionally successful in California[5].

BayBio also spends considerable time crafting press releases, working with various media outlets, as well as sponsoring conferences and workshops to cultivate the entrepreneurial spirit of biotechnology. This spirit has been fed from deep pockets; from 1995 to 2001, the Bay Area, 'received 31% of all venture capital investments in biopharmaceuticals' (Le Merle and Michels 2003: 4). This influx of capital has increased the importance of BayBio as biotechnology booster. Like CAMR, BayBio orchestrates the linkages and infrastructural development requisite for the organised functioning of an economic sector. However, this work is also producing political effects, including a version of public space that is simultaneously 'doable' and ethical. This imagination implicates (Clarke and Montini 1993) PAGs and science movements as part of the field of biotechnology.

Conclusions: biotechnology and potentiality

As Pierre Bourdieu has argued, there are contests of structuring, distinction and exclusion that are at stake in any field. These are clearly important processes for the emergence of the (semi) autonomous fields that constitute social life. In this chapter I have looked at four movements that have stakes in the debates over ESC research. The point here is not to categorise these groups as either old or new social movements. Rather, this work has highlighted the ways in which they engage with a broad set of questions involving, in the words of Nikolas Rose, the politics of 'life itself' (Rose 2001). However, the constellations of positions and actors involved with biotechnology and biomedical research reveal different processes at work in the field from those Bourdieu considered important. In this chapter I have argued that the field of biotechnology also operates through the politics of *potentiality*.

Biomedical research and biotechnology constantly reshuffles the terrains of life and death via interventions through the beginning of life until well past senescence. The dispersion of time itself into a series of infinitesimal moments has allowed gametes, blastocysts and frozen embryos to become categorised as both persons and property. Here, citizen participation is facilitating the construction of a quasi-object that is also a quasi-subject (Latour 1993). Competing imagined futures represent competing conceptualisations of time. For Theresa at Snowflakes, frozen embryos fast-forward in the blink of an eye to become aunts and uncles, while for Stephanie and CAMR, the same frozen embryos dissolve back into a pre-embryonic ground state of cellular potential that will transform medicine.

Snowflakes and CAMR both contest the status of the frozen embryo. They deploy arguments, produce artefacts, and exert influence within the domains that they are active in. The analysis conducted here has argued that these different techniques and mechanisms become *political technologies* as they organise and classify, as well as bring to light, the possibilities of new relationships and subjectivities. A political technology does not just delimit or repress, but brings to vision the potential of a novel set of arrangements (Foucault in Faubion 2003: 403). Political technologies work not only within focal movements, but circulate between movements, and operate within a field.

A key aspect of the political technologies within the field of biotechnology is the cultivation of potentiality. This potentiality is important across scales. For example, it is part of the process of how actors come to inhabit a 'politicized collective illness identity' (Brown *et al.* 2004). These identities are a consequence of activist politics and embodied experience, but it is also at stake in larger debates about the consequences of ESC research. CAMR and BayBio are both deeply reliant upon these identities, and they are major components of the political imagination that each of these groups produces for very different outcomes.

This attention to the potentiality of fields builds on the work of both Bourdieu and Appadurai[6]. Bourdieu consistently called attention to the field-level effects of social interaction. While fields are crucial framing structures of social action, emphasis must also be placed on their permeability and mutability. These aspects of the field are generative of potentiality; in Appadurai's terms, it is the *imagined* aspects of identity and location that provoke the dynamic nature of fields. Appadurai has focused on the imagination as a key site for understanding emergent global forms: '[T]he imagination has become an organized field of social practices, a form of work (in the sense of both labor and culturally organized practice), and a form of negotiation between sites of agency (individuals) and globally defined fields of possibility' (Appadurai 1996: 31). Thus, by paying attention to the imagined, potential aspects of the field of biotechnology, Bourdieu's somewhat static depiction of a field can be extended.

This analysis has also demonstrated that there are multiple positions around the debates over ESC research. Eschewing a binary or 'pro/con' approach, and focusing on a field of relationships and conflicts, deepens understandings of how 'biomedicalization' is operating and transforming both biomedicine and the subjects that live and move within and across its uneven and stratified terrains (Clarke *et al.* 2003). This in turn offers new avenues to think about the ways in which actors participate in the construction of biomedical knowledge. Actors take part in social movements as patients, supporters/opponents and citizens, among other categories, and this field analysis has demonstrated how each of those categories is important in struggles over potential identities and futures.

Finally, this perspective invites a wider geographical perspective; while this work has focused on the United States, others have looked at how fields of biotechnology between and across nations are contiguous and/or disjunctive (for example, Bud 1993, Franklin and Lock 2003, Franklin *et al.* 2000, Gottweis 1998, Lock 2002, Rabinow 1999). While biomedical science and biotechnology have become international institutions, it is crucial to retain the specificity of how these institutions and practices contribute to the production of fields in relation to the historical conditions within which they are situated.

Acknowledgements

I would like to thank Phil Brown, Renée Beard, Cassandra Crawford, Adele Clark, Jennifer Fishman, David Hess, Nicholas King, Dale Rose and Stephen Zavestoski, as well as the anonymous reviewers for *Sociology of Health and Illness*, for insight and helpful criticism.

Notes

1 Testimony by JoAnn Davidson, 17th July 2001 before United States House of Representatives Subcommittee on Criminal Justice, Drug Policy, and Human Resources Hearing on Embryonic Cell Research (www.cmdahome.org).
2 Testimony by Marlene Strege, 17th July 2001 before United States House of Representatives Subcommittee on Criminal Justice, Drug Policy, and Human Resources Hearing on Embryonic Cell Research (www.cmdahome.org).

3   Fedex refuses to ship these items internationally: 'Human corpses, human organs or body parts, human and animal embryos, or cremated or disinterred human remains'. (www.fedex.com/us/services/express/termsandconditions/intl/prohibiteditems.html)

4   Other groups involved included the Bay Area Council and the Monitor group. The Bay Area Council was formed in 1945 and it mission is to 'sustain business leadership that fosters excellence in public policy to promote economic prosperity and quality of life in the Bay Area' (www.bayareacouncil.org). The Monitor Group is an umbrella corporation covering companies devoted to developing knowledge management techniques, integrated business systems and evaluation services for venture capital (www.monitor.com).

5   On 22 September 2002, California governor Gray Davis signed Senate Bill 253 into law, authorising both derivation and research on ESCs in California (Jones 2002).

6   I thank David Hess for pointing this out.

References

Aldhous, P. (2001) Can they rebuild us? *Nature*, 410, 622–25.

Anderson, W. (1998) Leprosy and citizenship, *Positions: East Asia Cultures Critique*, 6, 707–30.

Appadurai, A. (1996) *Modernity at Large: Cultural Dimensions of Globalization*. Minneapolis: University of Minnesota Press.

Arenas, E. (2002) Stem cells in the treatment of Parkinson's disease, *Brain Research Bulletin*, 57, 6, 795–808.

Becker, H. (1982) *Art Worlds*. Berkeley: University of California Press.

Benford, R. (1997) An insider's critique of the social movement framing perspective, *Sociological Inquiry*, 67, 4, 409–30.

Bonnicksen, A.L. (2002) *Crafting a Cloning Policy: from Dolly to Stem Cells*. Washington, DC: Georgetown University Press.

Borlongan, C. and Sanberg, P. (2002) Neural transplantation for treatment of Parkinson's disease, *Drug Discovery Today*, 7, 12, 674–82.

Bourdieu, P. (1975) The specificity of the scientific field and the social conditions of the progress of reason, *Social Science Information*, 14, 6, 19–47.

Bourdieu, P. (1990) *The Logic of Practice*. Palo Alto, CA: Stanford University Press.

Bourdieu, P. (1991) The peculiar history of scientific reason, *Sociological Forum*, 6, 1, 3–26.

Bourdieu, P. and Wacquant, L.J.D. (1992) *An Invitation to Reflexive Sociology*. Chicago: University of Chicago Press.

Brodwin, P. (2000) *Biotechnology and Culture: Bodies, Anxieties, Ethics*. Blooming-ton: Indiana University Press.

Brown, P., Zavestoski, S., McCormick, S., Mayer, B., Morello-Frosch, R. and Gaisor, R. (2004) Embodied health movements: uncharted territory in social movement research, *Sociology of Health & Illness*, 26, 1–31.

Brundin, P. and Hagell, P. (2001) The neurobiology of cell transplantation in Parkinson's disease, *Clinical Neuroscience Research*, 1, 507–20.

Bud, R. (1993) *The Uses of Life: a History of Biotechnology*. Cambridge: New York, Cambridge University Press.

Clarke, A. (1990) A social worlds research adventure: the case of reproductive science. In Cozzens, S.E. and Gieryn, T.F. (eds) *Theories of Science in Society*. Bloomington: Indiana University Press.

Clarke, A. and Gerson, E. (1990) Symbolic interactionism in social studies of science. In Becker, H.S. and McCall, M.M. (eds) *Symbolic Interaction and Cultural Studies*. Chicago: University of Chicago Press.

Clarke, A., Mamo, L., Shim, J., Fishman, J. and Fosket, J. (2003) Biomedicalization: technoscientific transformations of health, illness, and U.S. biomedicine, *American Sociological Review*, 68, 161–94.

Clarke, A. and Montini, T. (1993) The many faces of RU486: tales of situated knowledges and technological contestations, *Science Technology and Human Values*, 18, 1, 42–78.

Daley, G. (2002) Prospects for stem cell therapeutics: myths and medicines, *Current Opinion in Genetics and Development*, 12, 607–13.

Dobnik, V. (1998) Frozen for the future, thousands of embryos linger in legal oblivion, *Los Angeles Times*, 15th March 10. Los Angeles.

Dominguez-Bendala, J., Ricordi, C. and Inverardi, L. (2002) Stem cells and their clinical application, *Transplantation Proceedings*, 34, 1372–5.

Faubion, J.D. (ed.) (2000) *Michel Foucault: Power, Volume 3*. New York: The New Press.

Franklin, S. and Lock, M.M. (2003) *Remaking Life and Death: Toward an Anthropology of the Biosciences*. Santa Fe: School of American Research Press.

Franklin, S., Lury, C. and Stacey, J. (2000) *Global Nature, Global Culture*. London: Sage.

Fujimura, J. (1988) The molecular biological bandwagon in cancer research: where social worlds meet, *Social Problems*, 35, 261–83.

Fujimura, J.H. (1996) *Crafting Science: a Sociohistory of the Quest for the Genetics of Cancer*. Cambridge, Mass: Harvard University Press.

Gaudillière, J.-P. and Löwy, I. (1998) *The Invisible Industrialist: Manufactures and the Production of Scientific Knowledge*. New York: Macmillan Press.

Goodwin, J. and Jasper, J.M. (1999) Caught in a winding, snarling vine: the structural bias of political process theory, *Sociological Forum*, 14, 1, 27–54.

Goodwin, J., Jasper, J.M. and Polletta, F. (2001) *Passionate Politics: Emotions and Social Movements*. Chicago: University of Chicago Press.

Gottweis, H. (1998) *Governing Molecules: the Discursive Politics of Genetic Engineering in Europe and the United States*. Cambridge, Mass: MIT Press.

Guidry, J.A., Kennedy, M.D. and Zald, M.N. (2000) *Globalizations and Social Movements: Culture, Power, and the Transnational Public Sphere*. Ann Arbor: University of Michigan Press.

Heinberg, R. (1999) *Cloning the Buddha: the Moral Impact of Biotechnology* (1st Quest Edition). Wheaton, Ill: Quest Books.

Holland, S., Lebacqz, K. and Zoloth, L. (2001) *The Human Embryonic Stem Cell Debate: Science, Ethics, and Public Policy*. Cambridge, Mass, London: MIT Press.

Jasper, J.M. (1997) *The Art of Moral Protest: Culture, Biography, and Creativity in Social Movements*. Chicago: University of Chicago Press.

Jenkins, J.C. (1983) Resource mobilization and the study of social movements, *Annual Review of Sociology*, 9, 527–53.

Johnston, H. and Klandermans, B. (1995) The cultural analysis of social movements. In Johnston, H. and Klandermans, B. (eds) *Social Movements and Culture*. Minneapolis: University of Minnesota Press.

Jones, G. (2002) Bill boosting stem-cell research to be signed: Davis will OK measure that paves the way for government funding of the controversial work, *Los Angeles Times*, 22nd September. Los Angeles.

Kennedy, D. and Kallenbach, M. (1996) Couples rush to save their embryos, *The Times of London*, 1st August, Section 4M. London.

Kirejczyk, M.S.M. (2000) Users, values, and markets: shaping users through the cultural and legal appropriation of in vitro fertilization. In Saetnan, A.R., Oudshoorn, N. and Kirejczyk, M.S.M. (eds) *Bodies of Technology: Women's Involvement with Reproductive Medicine*. Columbus, OH: Ohio State University Press.

Klandermans, B. and Johnston, H. (1995) *Social Movements and Culture*. Minneapolis: University of Minnesota Press.

Klawiter, M. (1999) Racing for the cure, walking women, and toxic touring: mapping cultures of action within the Bay Area terrain of breast cancer, *Social Problems*, 46, 1, 104–26.

Krimsky, S. (1991) *Biotechnics and Society: the Rise of Industrial Genetics*. New York: Praeger.

Kroll-Smith, S. and Floyd, H.H. (1997) *Bodies in Protest: Environmental Illness and the Struggle over Medical Knowledge*. New York: New York University Press.

Latour, B. (1993) *We Have Never Been Modern*. Cambridge, Mass: Harvard University Press.

Le Merle, M. and Michels, N. (2003) Taking action for tomorrow: Bay Area life sciences strategic action plan, Sacramento, CA, Office of the Governor.

Lindvall, O. and Hagell, P. (2001) Cell therapy and transplantation in Parkinson's disease, *Clinical Chemistry and Laboratory Medicine*, 39, 4, 356–61.

Lock, M.M. (2002) *Twice Dead: Organ Transplants and the Reinvention of Death*. Berkeley: University of California Press.

MacKay, R. (2000) Stem cells – hype and hope, *Nature*, 406, 361–4.

McAdam, D. (1999) *Political Process and the Development of Black Insurgency, 1930–1970* (2nd Edition). Chicago: University of Chicago Press.

McAdam, D., Tarrow, S.G. and Tilly, C. (2001) *Dynamics of Contention*. New York: Cambridge University Press.

McCarthy, J. and Zald, M. (1977) Resource mobilization and social movements: a partial theory, *American Journal of Sociology*, 82, 1212–41.

Mulkay, M.J. (1997) *The Embryo Research Debate: Science and the Politics of Reproduction*. New York: Cambridge University Press.

Rabinow, P. (1996) *Making PCR: a Story of Biotechnology*. Chicago: University of Chicago Press.

Rabinow, P. (1999) *French DNA: Trouble in Purgatory*. Chicago: University of Chicago Press.

Rose, N. (2001) The politics of 'life itself', *Theory, Culture and Society*, 18, 6, 1–30.

Snow, D. and Benford, R. (1992) Master frames and cycles of protest. In Morris, A. and Mueller, C.M. (eds) *Frontiers in Social Movement Theory*. New Haven, CT: Yale University Press.

Snow, D., Rochford Jr., E.B., Worden, S. and Benford, R. (1986) Frame alignment processes, mobilization, and movement participation, *American Sociological Review*, 51, 4, 464–81.

Snyder, E. and Vescovi, A. (2000) The possibilities/perplexities of stem cells, *Nature Biotechnology*, 18, 827–8.

Stanworth, S. and Newland, A. (2001) Stem cells: progress in research edging towards the clinical setting, *Clinical Medicine*, 1, 5, 378–82.

Stoddart, R. (2003) Embryo adoption agreement, Nightlight Christian Adoptions. Fullerton, CA.

Strauss, A. (1978) A social worlds perspective. In Denzin, N.K. (ed.) *Studies in Symbolic Interactionism 1*. Greenwich, CT: JAI Press.

Strom, T., Field, L. and Ruediger, M. (2002) Allogeneic stem cells, clinical transplantation and the origins of regenerative medicine, *Current Opinion in Immunology*, 14, 601–5.

Swidler, A. (1986) Culture in action: Symbols and strategies, *American Sociological Review*, 51, 2, 273–286.

Sylvester, E.J. and Klotz, L.C. (1983) *The Gene Age: Genetic Engineering and the Next Industrial Revolution*. New York: Scribner.

Tarrow, S.G. (1998) *Power in Movement: Social Movements and Contentious Politics* (2nd Edition) Cambridge England, New York: Cambridge University Press.

Taylor, V. and Whittier, N. (1995) Analytical approaches to social movement culture: the culture of the women's movement. In Johnston, H. and Klandermans, B. (eds) *Social Movements and Culture*. Minneapolis: University of Minnesota Press.

Teich, A. (2002) AAAS and public policy: speaking softly and carrying a medium-sized stick, *Technology in Society*, 24, 167–78.

Thackray, A. (1998) *Private Science: Biotechnology and the Rise of the Molecular Sciences*. Philadelphia: University of Pennsylvania Press.

Thomson, J.A., Itskovitz-Eldor, J., Shapiro, S.S., Waknitz, M.A., Swiergiel, J.J., Marshall, V.S. and Jones, J.M. (1998) Embryonic stem cell lines derived from human blastocysts, *Science*, 282, 5391, 1145–7.

Valone, D.A. (1998) The changing moral landscape of human reproduction: two moments in the history of in vitro fertilization, *Mount Sinai Journal of Medicine*, 65, 3, 167–72.

Chapter 6

Uneasy allies: pro-choice physicians, feminist health activists and the struggle for abortion rights

Carole Joffe, Tracy Weitz and Clare Stacey

Introduction

While most health-related social movements consist of consumer groups mobilised against the biomedical establishment and/or the state, the 'Abortion Rights Movement' represents a particularly interesting case because of the involvement of both feminist activists and a segment of the medical profession. Although both groups share the same general goal – legal abortion – their alliance has over time been an uneasy one, and in many ways a contradictory one. This chapter will trace the activities of each group on behalf of legal abortion (before *Roe v. Wade*) and accessible abortion (after legalisation). We will show points of convergence as well as points of contention between the two groups. Specifically, we will highlight the tensions between the feminist view of abortion as a women-centred service, with a limited, 'technical' role for the physicians, and the abortion providing physicians' logic of further medicalization/professional upgrading of abortion services as a response to the longstanding marginality and stigmatisation of abortion providers.

We think it especially important to focus on the relationship between physician and feminist wings of the Abortion Rights Movement, because, with a few notable exceptions (Luker 1984, Garrow 1994), the former have been left out of discussions of abortion activism. The dominant social movement analyses of abortion typically focus on 'pro-life' vs. 'pro-choice' activists (McCarthy 1987, Ferree *et al.* 2002, Saletan 2003) or anti-abortionists (Blanchard 1994, Risen and Thomas 1998, Mason 2002, Maxwell 2002, Wagner 2003). Even leading sociological studies that focus exclusively on the pro-choice movement (*i.e.* Staggenborg 1991) tend to leave out physicians as key actors. Our argument is that only by noting the evolving relationships between these two crucial sets of actors can one fully understand the contemporary abortion rights movement.

We will further argue that the abortion situation, while unique in some respects, offers an interesting perspective on an aspect of health social movements more generally, namely the relationships that can evolve between 'dissident' physicians and their lay allies. Abortion represents an instance of a 'boundary movement' (Brown *et al.* 2004) in which not only have the boundaries between professionals and lay activists become blurred, but to a certain extent, these two groups have arguably over time changed places, with the physicians becoming more politicised and the lay activists more professionalised. We will point to three distinct phases in this relationship between doctors and lay activists: the first in which physicians were reluctant reformers in an often tense relationship with feminist activists; the second in which physician and lay activists came together in a relationship of mutual dependence during the development of the first-generation of legal abortion facilities; and the present moment, in which physicians themselves engage in grassroots work, helped to a considerable degree by prochoice feminists who are now themselves considerably 'bureaucratised'.

History of physician mobilisation around abortion

The physician campaign to criminalise abortion in the 19th century
The first instance in the United States of physician mobilisation around abortion was actually a campaign to criminalise the procedure. Until the beginnings of this campaign in the mid-19th century, abortion was largely unregulated in the US (Mohr 1978, Luker 1984, Petchesky 1984, Smith-Rosenberg 1985). Though a number of groups participated in this criminalisation campaign, physicians were the leading force. The American Medical Association (AMA), formed in 1847, quickly made the criminalisation of abortion one of its highest priorities, a move based not on moral objections to abortion, but rather because the issue served so well as the centre of the new organisation's professionalising project (Starr 1982). Because abortion provision in the 19th century drew so heavily on nurses, midwives and other 'irregular' healthcare providers, mobilisation around this issue provided a highly suitable vehicle to differentiate 'regular' or 'elite' physicians from the wide variety of other groups also making claims to be legitimate healthcare providers in that period (Mohr 1978, Luker 1984).

The goal of the AMA campaign, however, was not simply to ban all abortions. Rather, the ultimately successful AMA position was that physicians should control the terms under which any 'authorized' abortions took place. By 1880 all states had regulated abortion but many states continued to permit abortions when there was a threat to the life of the mother, or a serious threat to her health as determined by a physician (Mohr 1978).

Physician responses to the 'century of criminalization'
The major result of this physician-led campaign around abortion was a 'century of criminalization' (from 1880 until the 1973 *Roe v. Wade* decision) whose chief feature was a flourishing market of illegal abortion. This long period of illegal abortion in the US in turn has had important consequences for the issues under consideration in this chapter. The first of these is the legacy of the 'back alley abortionist' concerning mainstream medical circles. Similarly, the difficulties women experienced in obtaining an abortion before legalisation had helped shape the way that a generation of feminist activists had perceived the need for abortion to be controlled by women.

Those involved in performing abortions during this 'century of criminal-ization' were a very diverse group, who varied with respect both to their medical training, and to their motivations. Some of those providers were trained; others were not. Some were highly competent; others caused hun-dreds of thousands of injuries and thousands of deaths. Some performed illegal abortions because of immense compassion for women in a desperate situation; the motivation of others was greed. But in spite of the diversity of the actual universe of abortion providers in the pre-*Roe* era, it is the back alley 'butcher' or 'abortionist' (terms that have been used interchangeably) that has most strongly captured the imagination of the medical profession. The most egregious stories tell of men (some physicians, some not) who performed abortions in filthy settings, under the influence of alcohol, and who demanded sexual favours from their terrified and vulnerable patients (Messer and May 1988, Miller 1993) The figure of the abortionist came to symbolise a potent combination of professional ineptness, ethical lapses and, of course, an association with the controversial issues of sexuality and gender (Jaffe, Lindheim and Lee 1981, Joffe 1995). This aversion to the abortion provider – even while increasing support for legal abortion was growing within medical ranks – sets the stage for the considerable chal-lenges that would lie ahead for the medical wing of the abortion rights movement.

Physician experiences of illegal abortion
Throughout the era of criminalisation, US physicians faced an ambiguous, and increasingly, untenable situation vis-à-vis abortion. The state statutes that the AMA had so vigorously promoted did not make all abortions illegal; rather, as suggested above, they authorised the medical profession to decide which abortions would be authorised. But in many instances there was no uniform agreement on which conditions posed a true threat to the woman's life, or what degree of threat to her health merited an authorised abortion. As the work of Luker (1984) has shown, the medical profession in the years leading up to *Roe* split into two factions with respect to abortion: the 'strict constructionists', those morally opposed to abortion, who wanted their col-leagues to adhere to the most rigid interpretations of the laws governing authorised abortions, and the 'broad constructionists', who pushed for a far more expansive and discretionary interpretation of abortion policies.

The ambiguous nature of approved abortion created difficulties for physi-cians in practice in the 1950s and 1960s. Those who worked with women of reproductive age faced requests for abortions in a legal 'grey area' where it was often not entirely clear what constituted a 'legal' abortion and what did not. Moreover, as medical management of pregnancy improved throughout the 20th century, fewer and fewer of their patients qualified under the 'threat to life' or even 'health' guidelines (Luker 1984). In most American hospitals, abortion decisions were made informally, with inevitable tensions rising between the strict and the broad constructionists.

Even those doctors who did not directly deal with adult women in their professional practices typically had encountered in hospital emergency rooms, during their internship or residency periods, the ravages of illegal abortion. Women who were seriously injured, either as a result of attempted self-abortion, or at the hands of an inept practitioner, so overwhelmed hospital facilities in the pre-*Roe* era that some hospitals established special wards to care for them, sometimes referred to, sardonically, as 'septic tanks' (a reference to the life-threatening sepsis infections in the bloodstream that often resulted from illegal abortion). One respected estimate put the number of deaths from illegal abortions in the years leading up to *Roe* at 5,000 (Leavy and Kummer 1962). This situation of abortion in the decades before legalisation was instrumental in moving a generation of US physicians towards increasing discomfort with the status quo.

Abortion rights physicians begin to mobilise
Although there had been earlier discussions of legalising abortion within the medical profession, mobilisation around this issue began in earnest in the 1950s. Planned Parenthood, an organisation that had till then studiously avoided the abortion question, took the unprecedented step of hosting a conference on the subject in 1955 (Calderone 1958). Many sympathetic physicians of that era became involved shortly thereafter with the efforts of the American Law Institute (ALI), which in 1959 proposed a model abortion reform bill permitting the procedure on certain limited grounds (Garrow 1994). Abortion reform was framed as a desire to give expanded discretion to the medical profession (Stetson 2001). This initial physician interest in abortion law reform, rather than outright repeal of existing law, would shortly put them at odds with 1960s feminist activists.

In 1964, one of the first explicitly abortion-reform organisations, the Association for Humane Abortion [shortly to change its name to the Association for the Study of Abortion (ASA)] was founded in New York by a mixed group of physicians and laypeople. The group very deliberately elected a physician, Robert Hall, as its head, because of the belief that 'the future of the organization can best be served by a physician in the role of chairman' (Garrow 1994: 297). In 1968 the ASA hosted an international conference on abortion in Hot Springs, VA at which US physicians were exposed for the first time to the vacuum suction machine, a new technology for performing first trimester abortions that was considerably safer than the previously-used technique of dilation and curettage (D&C) (Hall 1970a).

Two key events occurred in the 1960s that further moved both the general public and the medical profession, respectively, in favour of legalised abortion. The first was the case of Sherri Finkbine, a well-known children's television personality in Phoenix. In 1962 Finkbine, while pregnant with her fifth child, took thalidomide, a drug she shortly learned was strongly associated with severe birth defects. Because of the public nature of her case, she was unable to arrange a legal abortion in Arizona and ultimately went to

Sweden to have an abortion. The case received widespread attention in the national media, and was instrumental in alerting the public about the diffi- culties of obtaining an abortion in a situation – e.g. a high likelihood of birth defects – that many Americans found justified the procedure (Luker 1984).

The second event – the case of the 'San Francisco Nine' – occurred in 1966 and involved nine San Francisco obstetrician/gynecologists who were abruptly threatened by the California Board of Medical Examiners with the loss of their medical licences because they had been performing abortions in local hospitals on women who had been exposed to rubella (German measles), which was also associated with birth defects. The case, however, had an unintended effect, in that it galvanised the members of the medical community, both in San Francisco and nationally, to defend their colleagues. This defence of the accused physicians can be explained by their professional stature (all held positions in prestigious local medical institutions) – unlike the infamous back alley abortionists of the day who did not receive medi- cine's support when they faced criminal charges (Lader 1973, Garrow 1994). Leading figures from the medical community, joined by prominent citizens in law and other fields, formed a defence committee to pay their legal expenses. Most noteworthy, over two hundred physicians from across the country, including the deans of 128 medical schools, signed an amicus brief that was filed on their behalf (Joffe 1995, Dynak et al. 2003).

Both the Finkbine and the SF-Nine case did not concern the rights of women to end an unwanted pregnancy, but rather the issue of fetal deform- ities (Hull and Hoffer 2001). These abortions, called 'therapeutic abortions' to distinguish them from abortions for other reasons, had greater support among both physicians and the general public. However, growing requests for other abortions not meeting these explicit criteria continued to grow, and by 1970, the cumulative effect of all of the above-mentioned events further pushed many in the medical profession to join the larger social movement to legalise abortion, and to repudiate the limited reforms represented by the ALI proposal. Many of these pro-choice physicians became involved in campaigns then underway to legalise abortion in various states, including New York, which narrowly passed such legislation in 1970. Also in that year, the AMA at its annual meeting voted in favour of legal abortion, thereby reversing its campaign of some 100 years earlier to criminalise the procedure.

The discussion at that meeting, however, foreshadowed some of the prob- lems to occur in the future relationship between abortion rights physicians and feminist pro-choice activists. The first of these was the challenge to the traditional relationship between doctor and patient that resulted from the demedicalization of the abortion procedure. As one doctor said at the AMA gathering, 'Legal abortion makes the patient truly the physician: she makes the diagnosis and establishes the therapy' (Jaffe, Lindheim and Lee 1981: 67). Similarly, even physicians deeply committed to legal abortion voiced hesitation about what legal abortion would imply about the role of the physician in this new health service. As Robert Hall said, in a statement that was to prove quite prophetic, 'When it comes to the doctor, I think he is eventually going to be no more than a technician. This may be humiliating to him. But it is his unavoidable plight if we are to grant women their inherent right to abortion' (Hall 1970b: 109).

Reflecting these concerns, the AMA resolution that was passed by its House of Delegates contained the statement that doctors should not provide abortions 'in mere acquiescence to the patient's demand' (American Medical Association House of Delegate 1970: 388), a more conservative position than many of the most committed pro-choice physicians of the era (Halfmann 2003). Halfmann argues that the AMA passed the 1970 resolution because the group did not perceive legal abortion as a threat to doctors' material interest and only a minimal threat to their clinical autonomy. The AMA position framed abortion reform as a way to ensure professional autonomy and was at odds with the vision of feminist abortion rights groups mobilising on behalf of women's rights.

This frame of professional autonomy was reflected in the very language of the *Roe v. Wade* decision itself, further contributing to the uneasy relations between medicine and feminist activists. Justice Harry Blackmun, the chief author of the decision, had spent considerable time as counsel to the Mayo clinic, and in the eyes of observers (Garrow 1994, Reagan 1997), this experience led to a decision that stressed the prerogatives of the medical profession, rather than the 'rights' of women. Leading constitutional scholars including Lawrence Tribe (1985) and Ruth Bader Ginsburg (1985) have noted with concern the privileging of the physician within the *Roe* decision. As the *Roe v. Wade* [410 US 113 1973] decision reads:

> The decision vindicates the right of the physician to administer medical treatment according to his professional judgment up to the points where important state interests provide compelling justifications for intervention. Up to those points, the abortion decision in all its aspects is inherently, and primarily, a medical decision, and basic responsibility for it must rest with the physician (1973: 166).

The feminist critique of the *Roe* decision, however, goes beyond a simple critique of the role of physician authority, it also includes a questioning of the privacy basis for the decision. Privacy is a negative right, *e.g.* 'freedom from' intervention rather than a positive rights approach which ensures 'freedom to' something. This distinction would become meaningful as future court cases would find that women do not have the actual right to get an abortion, only the right to choose an abortion. Thus, the State is not obliged to pay for abortion or to ensure that one is available for women. Feminists' expansive view of abortion rights would come into conflict with the rights of physicians to not perform abortion, a power that they would use extensively as abortion became more controversial (Halfmann 2003).

The disengagement from abortion after Roe v Wade

In 1972, in anticipation of the imminent legalisation of abortion, one hundred professors of obstetrics and gynaecology (ob/gyn) published an open letter to their colleagues calling for an equitable sharing of the anticipated abortion patient load (AJOG 1972). Estimating (accurately) that there would be about one million abortions requested in the first year after legalisation, the statement confidently predicted, 'If only half the 20,000 obstetricians in this country do abortions, they can do a million a year at a rate of two per physician per week' (AJOG 1972: 992). In sharp contrast to this statement, however, the period after *Roe* is noteworthy for what did *not* occur within medical institutions. With the exception of a few organisations such as the American College of Obstetricians and Gynecologists (ACOG) and the American Public Health Association (APHA), medical organisations did not establish standards for abortion care, resident education bodies in the field of ob/gyn did not mandate abortion training, most hospitals did not establish abortion services (Jaffe Lindheim and Lee 1981) and nowhere near half of all practising ob/gyns took up abortion care after *Roe*. The reluctance of so many medical institutions and individual physicians to engage with abortion can best be understood as a reaction to the legacy of the pre-*Roe* era, and especially the stigma associated with the illegal abortionist.

Several factors, including this hands-off approach to abortion on the part of the medical community, came together in the 1970s to facilitate the development of the 'freestanding clinic', which remains to this day the predominant form of abortion delivery in the US (Henshaw and Finer 2003). These clinics had been pioneered in Washington, DC and in New York City, places that had legalised abortion several years before *Roe*, and to which women came from all over the country. The model reflected an uneasy collaboration between abortion-sympathetic physicians and feminist pro-choice activists who sought an alternative model for the provision of healthcare. The clinic model was facilitated by several technological advances of that period, including the introduction of the vacuum suction machine into US medicine and reliable means of local anaesthesia which meant that abortions could be safely and comfortably delivered outside a hospital. This model not only lowered the cost of the procedure, but also meant that staff could be selectively hired who were abortion supporters. The clinics have amassed an excellent safety record and continue today to offer abortion care at remarkably low cost (Grimes 1992). An unintended consequence of the success of the freestanding clinic, however, is that abortion care has become further marginalised from mainstream medicine. The existence of the clinics arguably helped relieve many abortion-sympathetic physicians from the perceived burden of becoming an abortion provider themselves (Joffe 1995).

Responding to the anti-abortion movement

A newly energised anti-abortion movement began a wide-ranging campaign in response to the *Roe v. Wade* decision. Anti-abortion legislators won numerous successes at both the state and federal levels in regulating abortion provision; an early and significant victory was the passage in 1976 of the Hyde amendment, which prohibited the use of Medicaid funds to pay for abortions. Because so few physicians were offering abortion, they did not represent a large enough constituency to mobilise the professional medical community to address this policy change.

Over the next two decades, abortion providers became bound by myriad state laws governing their practice, including biased information requirements, waiting periods, parental involvement, bans of use of public funds or facilities, facilities requirements, reporting mandates, and abortion procedure bans. These regulations have no analogue elsewhere in medicine. Most challenges to these regulations have been rejected despite the long safety record of outpatient abortion and the lack of proof that such regulations improve patient care, safety, or health (Centre for Reproductive Rights 2003).

In addition to growing regulation of abortion, a grassroots anti-abortion movement began aggressively to confront abortion patients and providers at abortion facilities. Throughout the 1980s, there were rising incidents of clinic blockades and sieges, vandalism, firebombings, harassment and stalking of providers at their homes as well as workplaces (Risen and Thomas 1998, Feminist Majority Foundation 2003, National Abortion Federation 2003). In 1993, David Gunn, a doctor in Florida who was shot as he entered a clinic, became the first abortion provider to be murdered by an anti-abortion extremist. To date (Autumn 2003), six additional members of the abortion-providing community have been killed and thousands more terrorised. It is now routine for abortion providers to wear bulletproof vests, and for clinics to resemble armed fortresses, with thick walls and constant video surveillance.

By the late 1980s, the combination of the historically-marginalised status of abortion provision and the upsurge in violence by the anti-abortion movement created an evident crisis in the supply of abortion providers. From 1984 to the present, the number of abortion providers continued to decline and currently there are fewer than 2,000 identifiable abortion providers (Finer and Henshaw 2003). Some clinics found that they had to rely on flying in doctors from elsewhere in the country to provide these services. Local doctors, even if sympathetic to abortion, found that they would become pariahs in their local medical communities if they provided abortion (Gorney 1989, Joffe 1995). Some clinics reported that they were simply unable to find enough doctors to staff an abortion service at all.

In response to these developments, the National Abortion Federation (NAF), the major professional association for abortion providers in North America, and ACOG jointly organised a 1990 symposium, 'Who will provide abortions?'. Various speakers, who were long-time providers and observers of abortion work, confirmed not only the nation-wide problem of a provider shortage, but also the low status of this work in the eyes of many medical professionals. They cited the perception of abortion work as tedious and unchallenging, even among those who were ideologically committed to it (National Abortion Federation 1991). Participants also focused on the failure to routinise abortion training into ob/gyn residency programmes after *Roe v Wade*. The normal mechanism by which such training would have become required – adoption by the Committee on Residency Education in Obstetrics and Gynecology (CREOG) – had never taken place. The final report of the symposium called for ob/gyn residencies to mandate training in first and second trimester abortion techniques. Recognising that many ob/gyns would continue not to provide abortion care, the Symposium also called for the use of mid-level health professionals – physician assistants, nurse midwives, nurse practitioners – to perform first trimester abortions, under physician supervision. As a result of this Symposium and follow-up work by attendees, CREOG for the first time in 1995 passed a resolution mandating routine training. In an unprecedented intrusion into medical accreditation activity, Congressional anti-abortion legislators quickly moved to nullify this action by CREOG, by passing a resolution stating that no residency programmes would lose federal funding if they did not comply with the new training requirements (Gray 1995).

As the violence and harassment against abortion providers intensified in the 1990s, countermovements (Lo 1982) arose among previously unaffiliated physicians and medical students. Medical Students for Choice (MSFC) formed in the summer of 1993 in direct response to the killing of Dr. Gunn and the mailing of a vulgar and threatening pamphlet about abortion providers to US medical students by Life Dynamics, an anti-abortion group in Texas (Joffe, Anderson and Steinauer 1998). MSFC spoke out forcefully for the need to incorporate material on abortion into medical school curricula as well as the need for greater protection of abortion providers (Hitt 1998). Shortly thereafter, a group of physicians in New York founded a national organisation, Physicians for Reproductive Choice and Health (PRCH). Unlike NAF, a group composed almost exclusively of abortion providers, PRCH is composed of abortion doctors as well as physicians committed to supporting abortion providers and addressing their long-standing stigmatisation. PRCH sought to include in its membership physicians with recognised authority in the medical profession, such as leaders of medical societies, renowned researchers, and academic chairs and deans.

Finally, efforts have been undertaken to institutionalise abortion training and research within mainstream medical institutions. With the help of a private donor, the Kenneth J. Ryan Residency Training Program in Abortion and Family Planning was established in 1999 to offer financial and technical support for ob/gyn residencies committed to establishing abortion training. The same donor has also funded a postgraduate Fellowship in Abortion and Family Planning. The intent of these programmes is to assure an abortion presence at leading medical schools in the United States, and to facilitate a new generation of physician researchers committed to a career in various facets of abortion care.

More recently, a group of family practice doctors, mostly centred in New York City, has organised to form the Access Project, which is committed to bringing abortion training to family practice and other primary care physicians. This group has worked assiduously to have abortion training incorporated into residency programmes other than those in ob/gyn. The Access Project's leaders have also mounted what can only be called a political campaign to persuade some reluctant leaders within family practice to allow abortion-relevant material at professional meetings and in the specialty's professional journals. The following fragment of an e-mail, sent by one of the leaders of the Access Project (and received by one of the authors) conveys the flavour of this group: 'What a great meeting we had last night in Boston! There were about 30 of us, from as far as Maine and Rhode Island, gathered together to figure out how to offer medical abortion in their practice sites. . . . The meeting provided such a great sense of . . . solidarity around working to overcome the barriers. . . .' (Anonymous 2002a).

In sum, the response of medical activists to the twin crises of provider shortages and anti-abortion harassment has been to counter the historic marginality of abortion provision. The activities listed above share the same goal of the integration of abortion care into mainstream medicine. Once again, abortion is at the core of a professionalising project for physicians. Unlike their 19th-century predecessors, however, contemporary physicians involved with abortion often engage in 'high-risk activism' (Taylor and Raeburn 1995), allied closely to feminist activists in the ongoing movement to secure abortion rights. Such effort, however, is ongoing within the changing context of healthcare in the US, in which physicians as a whole find that they have less authority. Increasingly, for-profit healthcare organisations run by administrators rather than physicians are the major political force behind healthcare policy. The reduction in physician dominance is exacerbated for the already marginalised abortion providers. In October 2003, the US Congress passed the so-called Partial Birth Abortion Ban, yet another unprecedented intrusion on the rights of physicians to practice medical care in accordance with their assessment of the needs of their patients (Stolberg 2003). In fighting this new law, as well as other limitations on practice, abortion providers look mainly to their feminist pro-choice allies, rather than to the healthcare system for support.

History of feminist involvement

Feminist health activists of the 1960s and 1970s

The earliest groups that had organised the mid-20th century on behalf of legalised abortion in the US were composed mainly of elite physicians, and their supporters from within the law, public health and other professional groups. As such, these groups operated in a quite staid, non-confrontational manner. Both the substance and style of abortion mobilisation changed dramatically in the 1960s with the emergence of the 'second wave' of American feminism. Unlike the 19th century US feminist movement (Gordon 2002), women's health generally, and abortion rights in particular, were key concerns of the second wave feminist movement (Ruzek 1978, Petchesky 1990, Rosen 2000, Morgen 2002). Similar to other oppositional healthcare movements of the 1960s, the women's health movement was concerned with the demystification of medical knowledge, bringing healthcare as much as possible under the control of patients, and changing the physician-patient relationship (Weisman 1998). But the unique aspect of the feminist health movement was its critique of medicine in 'patriarchal' terms. Ob/gyn, the subspecialty of medicine most concerned with adult women, and the male ob/gyn, were subjected to particular scrutiny by the women's health activists and came to symbolise for some feminists of that period all that was wrong with medicine, and indeed, with men's power over women (Ehrenreich and English 1978). As Starr (1982), commenting on the healthcare movements of the 1960s and 1970s, has observed, 'Perhaps nowhere was the distrust of professional domination more apparent than in the women's movement' (1962: 381, see also Epstein 1996).

Feminist activists in the field of abortion worked simultaneously on two fronts: making abortion legal, and helping women gain access to safe illegal abortions in the meantime. But though ostensibly joined with the physicians of that era who had similar goals, feminist activists were dismayed at the former's acceptance of reform – rather than outright repeal – of abortion laws. Moreover, the tactics used by feminist groups in that period were quite different from those used by physician groups.

In New York State, feminist demonstrations at legislative hearings and courtrooms were frequent. One of the best known of such actions was the disruption of a 1969 New York State legislative hearing by a recently formed 'radical feminist' group, the Redstockings. The group was enraged that the witness list of this hearing included 14 men and only one woman – a Roman Catholic nun. In a pattern that was to become familiar, the feminists were denounced by the mainstream pro-choice forces present, as well as those opposed to abortion (Garrow 1994). Other similar events took place in courtrooms where abortion was under discussion. For example, three feminist lawyers wrote of the courtroom atmosphere in 1969, where an early challenge to New York abortion law was being heard, 'It was a fun demonstration, something other movements have been using all along. A substantial number of women came to court and brought two things with them: babies, crying babies, and coat hangers. When they left, they took the babies along with them but left the coat hangers scattered all over the courtroom' (Goodman, Schoenbrod and Stearns 1973). One observer, writing of the period leading up to the New York law, spoke of pro-choice legislators' dismay at the 'counterproductive "strident" demonstrations and public testimony by militant feminists' (Moore 1971: 17).

The Jane collective, established in Chicago in 1969, was perhaps the most famous of the feminist-related abortion activities of the pre-*Roe* period; certainly it is the one that best captures the profound disconnect between the medical and feminist wings of the abortion rights movement of that period. The collective was a group of women, mostly in their twenties, who were connected to the leading local feminist group, Chicago Women's Liberation Union. The group initially operated an underground abortion service, making use of a provider whom they thought was a physician. The abortions took place in members' apartments and members of the collective assisted in the procedure. The name Jane was used in response to all phone calls, both as a security measure and as affirmation of the group's communal identity (Kaplan 1995). Upon finding out that their provider was not in fact a physician, some members of the collective asked to be taught by him and became providers themselves. The collective operated until 1973, when *Roe v. Wade* made their services no longer necessary. The group performed about 11,000 abortions in all, with no fatalities, and only one serious confrontation with the police (Garrow 1994, Kaplan 1995, Reagan 1997). The Jane collective attained legendary status within some sectors of the women's health community, not only for its bravado, but also for its demonstration that abortions could be done by women for women – in short, abortion could be demedicalized.

It was thus an atmosphere of wariness, if not distrust, in which abortion rights physicians and feminist health activists came together to form the first freestanding clinics in New York state and Washington, DC, both of which had legalised abortion before *Roe*. Some of the clinics of this era were established as for-profit ventures, others were nonprofit enterprises, with a physician acting as medical director, but a lay person as executive director, and a board consisting of both medical and nonmedical members. It was in these clinics that the new occupational role of 'abortion counselor' was developed (Joffe 1986). As an early edition of *Our Bodies, Ourselves* (1973), the preeminent document of the women's health movement stated, in a section written for those considering abortion, 'Probably the most important person you would come in contact with during an abortion would be the abortion counselor' (Boston Women's Health Book Collective 1973: 147).

These counsellors were typically women who had worked in the abortion rights movement, and who often themselves had undergone an illegal abortion. Their role was to advocate for the patient, which meant both explaining the technical aspects of the abortion procedure, accompanying her throughout the process, and intervening on her behalf, if she had any difficulties during her stay at the clinic, including difficulties with the attending physician. Thus, the counsellors monitored the doctors carefully, to make sure they were not causing undue pain and also that they were treating patients and staff with due respect. As a counsellor in one of the first New York clinics reminisced, some years later, about those heady first months of clinic operations:

It blows my mind, thinking about it now, about how much power we [the counsellors] had . . . The doctors were just terribly nervous about the whole thing and were willing to listen to us – about what kinds of counseling services there should be, lots of things. If one of the doctors they hired was causing too much pain or saying disgusting things to patients, we'd run into the director's office and get him fired. Unfortunately, the honeymoon period didn't last too long though (Joffe 1986: 36).

Besides their work in clinics, feminists in that period set up abortion referral services, which involved visiting the various clinics emerging after legalisation, and making their recommendations – both positive and negative – widely available through movement networks. The costs of abortion in the different facilities were of key concern to the feminist investigators, as was the quality of the physicians. In one well-publicised event, feminist activists sat in the lobby of one New York area clinic and handed patients leaflets stating the quality of services there was poor, and offered a list of recommended facilities (Ruzek 1978).

From the doctors' perspective, participation in such a different kind of medical setting could be very challenging, despite their commitment to legal abortion. Some male doctors (and most providers were male at that time) resented the covert, and sometimes overt, tone of 'male bashing' that they sensed from some of the counsellors. One male veteran of the early days of the freestanding clinics recalled that he felt very isolated from both the rest of the (female) staff and from the patients themselves, who were counselled either by nurses or lay counsellors. As he put it, 'I felt like a fool at the end of the curette' (Joffe 1995: 148). But even some women doctors found working in this new environment difficult, at least initially. Jane Hodgson, an ob/gyn in private practice for many years in Minnesota, worked at one of the first freestanding clinics in Washington in the early 1970s; her commitment to legal abortion was such that she put her licence in Minnesota in jeopardy by openly challenging that state's abortion laws in a test case (Garrow 1994). Nevertheless, she recounted her Washington experience, 'I'd never worked in a clinic. I'd always had my own practice and run my own show. I was not accustomed to counselors participating in medical decisions. . . . They had music playing all the time during procedures, very casual, no uniforms . . .' (Joffe 1995: 19).

To be sure, not every doctor who worked in the clinics in the years immediately surrounding *Roe* reported such difficulties. And both the doctors mentioned above went on to work for many satisfying years in such clinics. But whether the encounters were tense or pleasant, the point is that in the earliest years of legal abortion, there was a mutual dependency between physicians and activists. Activists needed the doctors, in most fundamental terms, because *Roe v. Wade* and subsequent decisions had made clear that abortions could not be performed by anyone other than a physician. But the doctors needed the feminists as well because the medical community as a whole had no idea what it meant to deliver abortion legally, in outpatient settings, to a large group of healthy women. The prior experience of most abortion-providing physicians, it should be recalled, was caring for women with serious health issues in a hospital setting, with an abortion performed under general anaesthesia. This first generation of feminist activists helped establish how outpatient abortion was to be done – for example, what kind of pre- and post-abortion counselling was needed – and also served as an important source of referrals for women flying in from all over the country. As such, clinic-based abortion further blurred the boundaries between lay and professional activist communities (Brown *et al.* in press). Doctors and women's health advocates worked together in a context where neither professional autonomy, nor activist ideology, reigned supreme. This uneasy alliance was born out of a commitment to provide women safe access to abortion, but ultimately demanded more: both doctors and feminists had to negotiate the lay/professional divide.

1980 to the present: the bureaucratisation of the pro-choice movement
After the *Roe* victory, like the larger women's movement of which it was a part, the feminist abortion rights movement gradually changed from being primarily a collection of local grass roots activist groups to coalescing into several larger 'social movement organisations' (SMOs) (Staggenborg 1991, Ferree and Martin 1995, Ruzek and Becker 1999). NARAL ProChoice America, originally founded in 1969 as the National Association for the Repeal of Abortion Laws, became the dominant single-issue group in the US dedicated to abortion (Garrow 1994). Other SMOs connected to the feminist movement, such as the National Organization for Women (NOW) and the Feminist Majority, though they work on a variety of issues, are heavily involved with abortion-related issues. These groups function with paid staffs, with Washington, DC headquarters (and in many instances, state and local chapters) and are sustained by a combination of membership dues, and large individual and foundation fund raising. The staff operate as Washington insiders, developing relationships with sympathetic politicians (Staggenborg 1991). The organisation's membership is mobilised to take various actions – such as writing to Congressional representatives and participating in voter registration drives, largely through mail, faxes and e-mail. One of these SMOs' remaining sixties-style activities is periodically to summon their membership, and the public at large, to huge marches in Washington to protect legal abortion. These marches are traditionally orderly and focus on protecting the *Roe v. Wade* decision.

While many women joined the early pro-choice feminist social movement out of their experience with illegal abortion, young women today, especially recent college graduates, typically join these SMOs through internships and entry-level employment. In contrast to the earlier generation, who engaged in civil disobedience and other forms of direct action, these new recruits are often assigned administrative tasks. As the authors heard one such young employee complain at a meeting, 'I joined the movement to make a difference and all I've been allowed to do is paste labels' (Anonymous 2002b).

To the extent that grass roots activism still exists in pro-choice circles, it is mostly at the site of clinics, where local groups have organised 'clinic defense' operations and 'escorting' of patients in response to anti-abortion disruptions. Though in most cases this support is highly welcomed by the clinic administration, it can at times be problematic, as some clinic defenders respond too emphatically to their opponents. One clinic manager said to one of the authors, 'A 15-year-old coming to the clinic, hearing all the screeching – she doesn't know or care if it's our side, or antis – she's just terrified' (Anonymous 1999).

A marked change in both rhetoric and style has accompanied this shift to more formalised organisational forms. 'Doctor bashing' and calls for 'demedicalized', 'woman-controlled' abortions are largely absent from contemporary abortion rights circles. (Indeed, somewhat ironically in light of the past, some of the major pro-choice organisations use the occurrence of anti-abortion attacks on doctors as part of their fundraising appeals.) This discursive shift is, of course, partly a reflection of the journey from '60s radical' to 'movement bureaucrat' or 'femocrat' undertaken by many feminist activists (Booth 1998). The less incendiary rhetoric also reflects that political culture more generally now in the United States is less receptive to such language – including, we might add, the donors on whom these SMOs rely for survival. But this retreat also reflects profound changes in the abortion landscape. First, there has been a huge increase in the number of women who have become doctors in the 30 years since the *Roe* decision (Morgen 2002), and a number of them have become abortion providers, thus blunting the earlier polarisation between the male doctor and the woman patient. Second, and most importantly, the combination of the shortage of abortion providers and the violence that abortion doctors have received at the hands of anti-abortion terrorists has made such rhetoric simply unfeasible.

Conclusion: accommodations and remaining contradictions

We suggest that there have been three distinct phases in the relationship of physicians and feminist activists: the first, in the years immediately preceding *Roe v. Wade*, where many abortion-sympathetic physicians were reluctant reformers, at odds not only with their colleagues but with feminists who had a far more expansive vision of abortion rights; the second, extending from the passage of *Roe* in 1973 until the early 1990s, where both parties existed somewhat tensely in a situation of mutual dependence; and the third, in which a far more activist group of doctors and their feminist supporters reached considerable accommodation with one another. The unanticipated strength and scope of the anti-abortion response to *Roe* has pushed these formerly uneasy allies into a tighter bond, in response to such a formidable opponent. Indeed, we can argue that as one observes the activities of each of these groups over time, it would appear that they have to a considerable degree blurred roles (Brown *et al.* 2004). Comparing the 1970s with the present, feminist supporters of abortion have changed in the direction of becoming less activist and more bureaucratic; physicians, on the other hand, have taken on the role of political activists within medicine.

But this increased activism among pro-choice physicians carries its own contradictions in several respects. First, activism on behalf of increased professionalism is inherently problematic – because professionalism and activism are viewed by many in medicine as incompatible with one another (Wynia *et al.* 1999) especially when the activism concerns such a contested social issue as abortion. Some of the pro-choice physicians who work energetically to promote abortion services and education within relevant medical organisations have told the authors of their concern that they are perceived by colleagues as 'fanatics' or 'single-issue types'.

Second, the professionalization agenda of pro-choice physicians is in conflict in key respects with the goal of increased abortion access. Nowhere is the conflict between these two goals more evident than in current developments around medication abortion. The preferred method for medication abortion involves the use of the mifepristone/misoprostol regime. Mifepristone, also known as RU-486 or the 'French abortion pill', was approved for use in the US in 2000 only after a protracted 12-year campaign mounted by both physician and feminist health activists. The legality of mifepristone was widely seen as an at least partial solution to the crisis in abortion access (Talbot 1999). Given that administering a drug requires less training than performing a surgical abortion, the pro-choice community hoped these new abortion technologies could both attract more providers, as well as integrate abortion provision into medical settings other than freestanding clinics, such as primary care practices (Talbot 1999). Immediately after approval of mifepristone by the Food and Drug Administration (FDA), pro-choice medical activists began an energetic round of trainings, across multiple primary care specialties. In particular, as discussed above, family practice doctors have lobbied heavily for inclusion of medication abortion in their residency programmes. And medication abortion has drawn considerable attention from advanced practice clinicians (APCs) – nurse practitioners, midwives, physician assistants – who see this form of abortion provision as squarely within their scope of practice. APCs are now providing medication abortion in a number of states, where this has been deemed legally permissible, and have formed their own organisation to promote such provision, Clinicians for Choice (2003).

But these medication abortion campaigns – while undeniably promoting access – nevertheless cut across the upgrading project of abortion providers. Medication abortion in several ways represents an instance of professional 'deskilling' (Haug 1973, Freidson 1984) by transforming abortion from a surgical procedure to the dispensing of a medication; by the claims that primary care physicians as well as specialists can safely provide abortion; and even more so, by the movement of APCs to become abortion providers. Additionally, medication abortion, far more than conventional vacuum aspiration abortion, puts more power in the hands of the patient herself. In the case of mifepristone, since the woman ingests the pills herself, it is arguably the woman who 'performs' the abortion. The provider, moreover, is dependent on the woman to comply with the rest of the regime, which involves inserting or ingesting the second medication, misoprostol, at home and returning to the clinic to ascertain that the abortion is complete. As research has shown, this transfer of agency to the patient is quite troubling to some contemporary providers (Simonds *et al.* 2001). Ironically, therefore, while this chapter has argued that feminist activists over time have largely accommodated changing political realities and given up old demands for 'woman-centred' abortion care, medication abortion, spurred on by physician activists, may well have the potential to resurrect this model.

What, finally, does the case of abortion described here have to tell us about physician/lay encounters in other health social movements? Abortion is in one sense unique because in no other contemporary case (or historical one for that matter) of a physician/lay movement does the former go to work in bullet proof vests; the extreme violence directed against abortion providers creates a dependence on lay allies in a way that is difficult to generalise to other situations. But in other ways the story told here does point to a promising stream of comparative research in other medical spheres where considerable social controversy exists, and therefore where both provider and patient risk stigmatisation. For example, both medical marijuana and physician-assisted suicide offer provocative cases with some key similarities to abortion. In both of the former, physicians often operate either in a grey area of legality (as did an early generation of pre-*Roe* abortion doctors) or in a situation of massive state regulation (as do contemporary abortion providers). Both of these fields have produced practitioners – 'dissident doctors' – who have become activists in the public arena, as well as within medical organisations (Quill 1993, Tuller 2003), and thus have incurred criticism from medical colleagues. Both of these fields moreover have generated intensely passionate lay adherents who have become knowledgeable about the medical components of their respective issues, and have also become sophisticated lobbyists.

Equally as significant, for the purposes of comparison, are the organised counter movements seeking to keep these activities illegal. And in the case of physician-assisted suicide, there may well be some echoes of the violence generated against abortion providers, given the opposition of the pro-life movement. In this regard, it is noteworthy that Randall Terry, the founder of one of the most militant anti-abortion groups, Operation Rescue, has surfaced as a major actor in one of the most high-profile 'right-to-die' cases in the US to date (Goodnough 2003). As researchers accumulate more case studies of health social movements in these and similar fields, we will presumably find a similar pattern of blurred boundaries between healthcare professionals and laypersons. Most particularly, the abortion story suggests that when dissident physicians become involved in arenas that are socially contested, they will find their strongest allies among lay activists, and may correspondingly jeopardise their standing among professional colleagues. Similarly, in contrast to an earlier generation of healthcare activists who sweepingly opposed 'medicine', contemporary activists will find it strategic, if not essential, to align with health professionals.

Acknowledgements

The authors would like to thank Fred Block, Drew Halfmann, Ann Hwang, the editors of this special issue and two anonymous readers for *Sociology of Health and Illness* for their comments on an earlier draft of this chapter. We would also like to thank Abigail Breckenridge for her excellent research assistance.

References

AJOG (1972) A statement on abortion by one hundred professors of obstetrics, *American Journal of Obstetrics and Gynecology*, 112, 7, 992–8.

American Medical Association House of Delegate (1970) American Medical Association: Annual Convention, Chicago, IL.

Anonymous (1999) Meeting Comment, 10 February.

Anonymous (2002a) Email, December.

Anonymous (2002b) Meeting Comment, October.

Blanchard, D.A. (1994) *The Anti-abortion Movement and the Rise of the Religious Right: from Polite to Fiery Protest*. New York, Toronto: Twayne Publishers, Maxwell Macmillan Canada.

Booth, K.M. (1998) National mother, global whore, and transnational femocrats: the politics of AIDS and the construction of women at the World Health Organization, *Feminist Studies*, 24, 1, 115–39.

Boston Women's Health Book Collective (1973) *Our Bodies, Our Selves: a Book by and for Women.* New York: Simon & Schuster.

Brown, P., Zavestoski, S., McCormack, S., Mayer, B., Morello-Frosch, R. and Gasior, R. (2004) Embodied health movements: new approaches to social movements in health, *Sociology of Health and Illness*, 26, 1–31.

Calderone, M.S. (ed.) (1958) *Abortion in the United States.* New York: Hoeber-Harper.

Centre for Reproductive Rights (2003) Targeted regulation of abortion providers: avoiding the 'TRAP' [Internet]. Available from: <http://www.crlp.org/pub_bp_trap.html> [Accessed 1 November, 2003].

Clinicians for Choice (2003) Clinicians for Choice: an organization of pro-choice nurse practitioners, midwives, and physician assistants [Internet]. Available from: <http://www.cliniciansforchoice.org/> [Accessed 30 June, 2003].

Dynak, H., Weitz, T.A., Joffe, C.E., Stewart, F.H. and Arons, A. (2003) *Celebrating San Francisco's Abortion Pioneers.* San Francisco, CA: Centre for Reproductive Health Research and Policy; University of California, San Francisco.

Ehrenreich, B. and English, D. (1978) *For her Own Good: 150 Years of the Experts' Advice to Women.* (1st ed) Garden City, NY: Anchor Press.

Epstein, S. (1996) *Impure Science: AIDS, Activism, and the Politics of Knowledge.* Berkeley: University of California Press.

Feminist Majority Foundation (2003) Monitoring clinic violence [Internet]. Available from: <http://www.feminist.org/rrights/clinicsurvey.html> [Accessed 30 June, 2003].

Ferree, M.M., Gamson, W.A., Gerhards, J. and Rucht, D. (2002) *Shaping Abortion Discourse: Democracy and the Public Sphere in Germany and the United States.* Cambridge, UK, New York: Cambridge University Press.

Ferree, M.M. and Martin, P.Y. (1995) *Feminist Organizations: Harvest of the New Women's Movement.* Philadelphia: Temple University Press.

Finer, L.B. and Henshaw, S.K. (2003) Abortion incidence and services in the United States in 2000, *Perspectives on Sexual and Reproductive Health*, 35, 1, 6–15.

Freidson, E. (1984) The changing nature of professional control, *Annual Review of Sociology*, 10, 1–20.

Garrow, D.J. (1994) *Liberty and Sexuality: the Right to Privacy and the Making of Roe v. Wade.* New York, Toronto: Macmillan Pub. Co.; Maxwell Macmillan Canada, Maxwell Macmillan International.

Ginsburg, R.B. (1985) Some thoughts on autonomy and equality in relation to *Roe v. Wade, North Carolina Law Review*, 63, 375.

Goodman, J., Schoenbrod, R.C. and Stearns, N. (1973) DOE and ROE: Where do we go from here? *Women's Rights Law Reporter*, 1, 4, 20–38.

Goodnough, A. (2003) Governor of Florida orders women fed in right-to-die case, *New York Times*, 22 October, A1, A20.

Gordon, L. (2002) *The Moral Property of Women: a History of Birth Control Politics in America.* 3rd Edition. Urbana and Chicago, IL: University of Illinois Press.

Gorney, C. (1989) Hodgson's choice: a long, cold abortion fight, *Washington Post*, 29 November, B1, B6-9.

Gray, J. (1995) Senate approves cutback in current federal budget, *New York Times*, 22 July, A7.

Grimes, D.A. (1992) Clinicians who provide abortions: the thinning ranks, *Obstetrics and Gynecology*, 80, 4, 719–23.

Halfmann, D. (2003) Historical priorities and the responses of doctors' associations to abortion reform proposals in Britain and the United States, 1960–1973, *Social Problems*, 50, 4, 567–9.

Hall, R.E. (ed.) (1970a) *Abortion in a Changing World*: Volume I, New York: Columbia University Press.

Hall, R.E. (ed.) (1970b) *Abortion in a Changing World*: Volume II, New York: Columbia University Press.

Haug, M.R. (1973) Deprofessionalization: an alternate hypothesis for the future, *The Sociological Review Monograph*, 20, 195–211.

Henshaw, S.K. and Finer, L.B. (2003) The accessibility of abortion services in the United States, 2001, *Perspectives on Sexual and Reproductive Health*, 35, 1, 16–24.

Hitt, J. (1998) Who will do abortions here? *New York Times Magazine*, 18 January, 20.

Hull, N.E.H. and Hoffer, P.C. (2001) *Roe v. Wade: the Abortion Rights Controversy in American History*, Kansas: Lawrence, KS, University Press.

Jaffe, F.S., Lindheim, B.L. and Lee, P.R. (1981) *Abortion Politics: Private Morality and Public Policy.* New York: McGraw-Hill.

Joffe, C. (1986) *The Regulation of Sexuality: Experiences of Family Planning Workers.* Philadelphia: Temple University Press.

Joffe, C. (1995) *Doctors of Conscience: the Struggle to Provide Abortion before and after Roe v. Wade.* Boston: Beacon Press.

Joffe, C., Anderson, P. and Steinauer, J. (1998) The crisis in abortion provision and pro-choice medical activism in the 1990s. In Solinger, R. (ed.) *Abortion Wars: a Half Century of Struggle, 1950–2000.* Berkeley: University of California Press.

Kaplan, L. (1995) *The Story of Jane: the Legendary Underground Feminist Abortion Service.* New York: Pantheon Books.

Lader, L. (1973) *Abortion II: Making the Revolution.* Boston: Beacon Press.

Leavy, Z. and Kummer, J.M. (1962) Criminal abortion: human hardship and unyielding laws, *Southern California Law Review*, 35.

Lo, C. (1982) Countermovements and conservative movements in the contemporary US, *Annual Review of Sociology*, 8, 107–34.

Luker, K. (1984) *Abortion and the Politics of Motherhood.* Berkeley: University of California Press.

Mason, C. (2002) *Killing for Life: the Apocalyptic Narrative of Pro-life Politics.* Ithaca, NY: Cornell University Press.

Maxwell, C.J.C. (2002) *Pro-life Activists in America: Meaning, Motivation, and Direct Action.* Cambridge, UK, New York: Cambridge University Press.

McCarthy, J.D. (1987) Pro-life and pro-choice mobilization: infrastructure deficits and new technologies. In Zald, M.N. and McCarthy, J.D. (ed.) *Social Movements in an Organizational Society: Collected Essays.* New Brunswick: Transaction Books.

Messer, E. and May, K.E. (1988) *Back Rooms: Voices from the Illegal Abortion Era.* New York: St. Martin's Press.

Miller, P.G. (1993) *The Worst of Times.* New York: Harper Collins.

Mohr, J.C. (1978) *Abortion in America: the Origins and Evolution of National Policy, 1800–1900.* New York: Oxford University Press.

Moore, E.C. (1971) Abortion and public policy: what are the issues? *New York Law Forum*, 17, 411–36.

Morgen, S. (2002) *Into our Own Hands: the Women's Health Movement in the United States, 1969–1990.* New Brunswick: Rutgers University Press.

National Abortion Federation (1991) *Who will Provide Abortions? Ensuring the Availability of Qualified Practitioners.* Washington: National Abortion Federation.

National Abortion Federation (2003) NAF violence and disruption statistics: incidents of violence and disruption against abortion providers in the US and Canada [Internet]. Available from: <http://www.prochoice.org/Violence/Statistics/stats.pdf> [Accessed 30 June, 2003].

Petchesky, R.P. (1984) *Abortion and Woman's Choice: the State, Sexuality, and Reproductive Freedom.* New York: Longman.

Petchesky, R.P. (1990) *Abortion and Woman's Choice: the State, Sexuality, and Reproductive Freedom, (Revised).* Boston: Northeastern University Press.

Quill, T.E. (1993) *Death and Dignity: Making Choices and Taking Charge.* New York: W.W. Norton.

Reagan, L.J. (1997) *When Abortion was a Crime: Women, Medicine, and Law in the United States, 1867–1973.* Berkeley: University of California Press.

Risen, J. and Thomas, J. (1998) *Wrath of Angels: the American Abortion War.* New York: Basic Books.

Roe v. Wade (1973) 410 US 113.

Rosen, R. (2000) *The World Split Open: how the Modern Women's Movement Changed America.* New York: Viking.

Ruzek, S.B. (1978) *The Women's Health Movement: Feminist Alternatives to Medical Control.* New York: Praeger.

Ruzek, S.B. and Becker, J. (1999) The women's health movement in the United States: from grass-roots activism to professional agendas, *Journal of the American Medical Women's Association*, 54, 1.

Saletan, W. (2003) *Bearing Right: how Conservatives Won the Abortion War.* Berkeley: University of California Press.

Simonds, W., Ellertson, C., Winikoff, B. and Springer, K. (2001) Providers, pills and power: the US mifepristone abortion trials and caregivers' interpretations of clinical power dynamics, *Health*, 5, 2, 207–31.

Smith-Rosenberg, C. (1985) The abortion movement and the AMA, 1850–1880. In Smith-Rosenberg, C. (ed.) *Disorderly Conduct: Visions of Gender in Victorian America.* New York: Knopf.

Staggenborg, S. (1991) *The Pro-choice Movement: Organization and Activism in the Abortion Conflict.* New York: Oxford University Press.

Starr, P. (1982) *The Social Transformation of American Medicine.* New York: Basic Books.

Stetson, D.M. (2001) *Abortion Politics, Women's Movements, and the Democratic State: a Comparative Study of State Feminism.* Oxford, UK, New York: Oxford University Press.

Stolberg, S.G. (2003) Senate approves bill to prohibit type of abortion, *New York Times*, 22 October, A1, A21.

Talbot, M. (1999) The little white bombshell, *New York Times Magazine*, 11 July, 38–43, 8, 61–3.

Taylor, V. and Raeburn, N. (1995) Identity politics as high risk activism: career consequences for lesbian, gay and bisexual sociologists, *Social Problems*, 42, 252–73.

Tribe, L.H. (1985) Commentary: the abortion funding conundrum: inalienable rights, affirmative duties, and the dilemma of dependence, *Harvard Law Review*, 99, 330.

Tuller, D. (2003) Doctors tread a thin line on marijuana advice, *New York Times*, 28 October, F5, F7.

Wagner, T.R. (2003) *Back to the Drawing Board: the Future of the Pro-life Movement.* South Bend, IN: St. Augustine's Press.

Weisman, C.S. (1998) *Women's Health Care: Activist Traditions and Institutional Change.* Baltimore, MD: Johns Hopkins University Press.

Wynia, M.K., Latham, S.R., Kao, A.C., Berg, J.W. and Emanuel, L.L. (1999) Medical professionalism in society, *New England Journal of Medicine*, 341, 21, 1612–6.

Chapter 7

Advocating voice: organisational, historical and social milieux of the Alzheimer's disease movement
Renée L. Beard

Introduction

Compared with the health social movements of other diseases, the Alzheimer's disease movement has been slow in identifying and implementing public spokespersons. Twenty-five years ago, practitioners and families working with and/or affected by Alzheimer's disease (AD) sought social change. When the first voluntary organisation was formed in its name, the intention was to direct attention to the condition and to garner financial support for research abetting a solution to AD. The movement successfully framed itself through the promotion of AD as a significant social, not simply individual, problem; transforming senility from a private family matter to a medical epidemic demanding public concern. The Alzheimer's disease movement illustrates the complexities involved in understanding the impact of external structures and internal dynamics on the maintenance, principles and outcomes of social movements and their organisations. The Alzheimer's Association, with (more recently) concerted effort from people with AD and (traditionally) their loved ones, has been a catalyst for the lobbying initiatives of the Alzheimer's movement. Despite intentions, attempts to give voice to the perspectives of people with AD have encountered considerable obstacles.

As with other marginalised groups, such as children, the learning disabled or the mentally ill, proxy interviews with carers have historically been seen as the best way to investigate issues of Alzheimer's disease; thus reinforcing the unfortunate notion that people with dementia are deficient. This view often stems from the belief that people with AD cannot learn or communicate in a meaningful way, do not want to, or would be harmed by the interaction. Such assumptions, created by and situated within a society that glamorizes a youthful, fit body and mind, further weaken the position of people with AD to assert their interests. In practice, the presumption of incompetence (Booth and Booth 1999) affects people with AD who cannot advocate for themselves, speak effectively in civic realms, or serve as leaders of the social movement claiming to represent them, regardless of their aptitude or aspirations. Ironically, the most salient barrier to challenging negative perceptions is precisely this lack of visible and credible spokespersons to portray the condition (Beard 2004). Understanding what impedes the Alzheimer's Association's attainment of certain objectives can inform the mobilisation efforts of other social movement organisations (SMOs), particularly those serving disadvantaged populations, trying to unify their constituents or incorporate spokespersons.

In the United States, the rise of activism in other arenas has proved that structural trends change when 'patient' advocates become visible, often forging new types of clinical research and practice (Epstein 1996, Fox and Mueller 2001, Klawiter 1999). The efforts of the AIDS and breast cancer movements were both critical of and galvanised biomedicine. These movements had large and ambitious groups of young, savvy, at-risk activists, including charismatic spokespersons, who generated urgency and support (Klawiter 1999, Kramer 1989) and could be effectively targeted for education and prevention; whereas the AD movement was not initiated by, or originally intended for, people with the condition. Further, since cognition is compromised with Alzheimer's, people are less likely (both presumptively and then in reality) to (be able to) advocate for themselves.

Historically, while the AIDS movement kept a local grassroots focus on individual needs, the AD movement's more macro national approach easily converted into an interest group aimed at making policy changes from within existing social structures (Rucht 1996). The Alzheimer's movement has not made concerted efforts to challenge medical authority or knowledge. In contrast, AIDS activism demanded drug trials and alternative therapies when no efficacious medications existed. The distinctions between these movements include the targeted populations (and their perceived aptitude) and goals regarding relations with and expectations of biomedicine.

The AD movement has been far more similar to the mental health and disability movements in terms of approaching biomedicine[1]. Despite a constituency comprising people with stated conditions, considerably fewer critical positions on biomedicine have surfaced in the mental health and disability movements than the AIDS or breast cancer movements. Arguably, this is due in part to the (once) historically contested legitimacy of certain conditions (*e.g.* mental illnesses) as a disease and/or the moral accountability often associated with physical disabilities (*e.g.* genetic deformities or weak immune systems). In addition, the perception of people with such conditions as vulnerable engenders an embittered struggle against assuming as a 'master status' the role of mentally ill/disabled person. The quest to be heard so feverishly achieved by these movements remains in elementary stages for people with AD. If the AD movement increasingly has components that do not embrace the biomedical model of Alzheimer's, then the resistance against the historical foundation of the Association will prove an important endeavour for people with AD in advocating their position.

The Alzheimer's Association – the countrywide powerhouse behind much of the movement in the US media, public discourse and research community – was established by care-providers and scientists. These underpinnings have yielded an impressive commitment to 'cause and cure' research, caregiver consequences, and long-term care policies. As diagnostic advancements identifying people in the earliest stages of AD, and even preclinically

(Golomb *et al.* 2001), have made it far more possible to obtain narrative accounts of Alzheimer's, the movement has begun to account for this phenomenon by trying to incorporate these voices instead of relying on the viewpoints of carers. Accordingly, the Association started altering their objectives as previously unheard perspectives emerged, including addressing new realms pertaining to quality of life, experiences of memory loss and meeting the individual needs of a diverse clientele. Traditional initiatives such as fundraising, education, family support and bench science are in direct competition for resources as attention shifts. As the largest and until very recently the only organisation aimed exclusively at dementia[2], the Association remains the most influential SMO in the AD movement. Discovering the factors influencing the activities of the Alzheimer's Association is essential to understanding what has frustrated the stated intentions of including people with AD.

Part of the obstacle to incorporating these perspectives may be due to the relationship between social death (Glaser and Strauss 1966, Kastenbaum 1969, Sudnow 1967), or marginalisation, and social worth. Research on dementia (Sweeting and Gilhooly 1997) suggests that those who suffer prolonged terminal illnesses, who are very old, and who are believed to experience a loss of personhood as a result of their condition are often relegated to inanimate objects. The symbolic liminality between life and death presumed of people with dementia risks rendering them socially obsolete. Such existential demarcations exacerbate the likelihood of societal disadvantages (Billis and Glennerster 1998) engendered by notions of AD as the 'never ending funeral' (Cutler 1986) and a 'living death' (Gubrium 1987). The 'competence-inhibiting support' (Booth and Booth 1999) implied by the surplus of manuals aimed at formal and informal providers of care signifies how easily those caring for people with AD become the object of attention and are often perceived as the second, if not the real, victims.

Although early attempts to incorporate the voice of people with dementia into research (Cohen 1991, Cottrell and Schulz 1993, Kitwood and Bredin 1992, Sabat and Harre 1992) did not gain necessary momentum, an impressive amount of both narrative accounts of Alzheimer's (Davis 1989, DeBaggio 2002, Dyer 1996, Henderson 1998, Friel-McGowin 1993, Rose 1996) and research that incorporates the perspective of people with AD (Braudy Harris 2002, Cheston and Bender 1999, Goldsmith 1996, Sabat 2001, Wilkinson 2002) has emerged. These studies have begun to reverse the trend of viewing people with AD primarily as confused, which pathologises their behaviour (Beard and Estes 2002, Bond 1992, Canguilhem 1991) and renders them effectively mute in public life.

Understanding the interface between cultures of media, politics and medicine and the efforts and obstacles of social movements and their organisations is crucial. If the objectives of the Association correlate with how clients or members are defined and treated, then the relations between SMOs and societal institutions have significant ramifications for people with AD. Societies tolerating age-based worth potentially stimulate institutional and structural forces that act to devalue, stereotype and exclude old people regardless of an SMO's intentions.

This research considers the ideological resources fuelling the Alzheimer's movement's central advocacy organisation and the milieux embedding it. Ideological differences create the issues around which social movements are initiated, objectives are delineated, constituencies are identified, and members are united. Biomedical definitions normalise, or name, diseases, thus making them a household word and legitimating their existence; naming illness serves to unite members of disease-based movements. Shifting the definition of Alzheimer's to include dementias of all ages circa 1975 greatly increased the number of reported cases and led to its being perceived as a significant social and health problem. The interrelationships between science, politics and cultures of disease have profound manifestations for members of health social movements, including the formation of collective identities, minimising blame-the-victim mentalities, influencing policy changes, procuring research monies and increasing awareness of targeted conditions.

The Association's dynamics impact not only upon people with dementia who may or may not be involved in the movement, but also all people with conditions where competence is questioned, such as children and those with mental illnesses, disabilities or brain disorders. Despite barriers, the increasing social movement involvement of people with AD continues to inform policy, practice and research. An examination of the Association's origins, ideology, goals and tactics can begin to address why incorporating this voice meets such resistance and can serve as a heuristic device for informing the mobilisation efforts of other SMOs.

Methods

These data are part of a larger research project informed by grounded theory and phenomenology. Data were gathered in a semi-structured manner with open-ended guides. Focus groups and interviews were conducted to collect detailed accounts of experiences with AD-diagnoses and of the philosophy of both individual staff members and the Association.

Sampling

The first part of the sample consisted of two one-hour focus groups (N = 12) and two-hour in-depth interviews (N = 6) with people diagnosed in the early stages of AD (ESAD). The elapsed time since diagnosis varied from weeks to years, since 'stage' refers to a categorisation independent of illness duration. All respondents were over 70 years old (mean = 73.5). There were 11 men and seven women. All but four were married and resided with a spouse: three (women) were widowed and one (man) was single, and all four lived alone. The focus groups were conducted at local Alzheimer's Association chapters in pre-existing support groups for people diagnosed with ESAD. The respondents for in-person interviews were recruited from the diagnostic centre of a large, research-based university in northern California.

The second component included a convenience/snowball sample to perform in-depth interviews with staff members (N = 12) of the Alzheimer's Association. All respondents had been with the Association for at least a year (mean = 4 years). There were five men and seven women. These respondents were representatives of Public Relations, Public Policy, Community Outreach, Development and Communication and Education/Program Management departments at eight chapters, both rural and urban, throughout the United States.

Data collection and analysis

Data from interviews and field notes were taped and transcribed. All data, including memos and textual materials, were then analysed using the constant comparative method and coding paradigm of grounded theory (Glaser and Strauss 1967, Corbin and Strauss 1998). The on-going process of taking notes, writing memos and reading data lends itself to emergent themes and categories for simplifying and articulating data. As coding occurred, themes emerged from the data; theory was inductively derived. The general principles of phenomenology (Schutz 1967) that highlight the subjective, lived-experiences of everyday life and illness experiences and the daily work performed by Association staff also informed this study. The main tools of this paradigm were the need for reflexivity, describing the structures of experience, and the constant reminder that subjectivity is processual and, therefore, data reflect a snapshot of the daily lives of the people in this study when they were interviewed.

Detailed notes were dictated promptly after each interview to ensure that emerging theoretical thoughts and a general overview of the data was recorded. Throughout the process, interviews were replayed or reread as soon as possible to encourage incremental development of theory and categorisation of ideas and themes. Analysis began with 'open coding' (Strauss and Corbin 1990) that involved identification of the dimensions and properties of the themes as they emerged. As more themes were discovered and the feeling of saturation occurred, themes were consolidated by using an explanatory matrix to identify 'core variables'; again, these themes were constantly verified as a tool of quality control.

The focus group occurred at the regularly scheduled time and place of the support groups. The interviews with people AD-diagnosed took place in their homes. Interviews with staff were performed both in-person at local chapters (N = 6) and by telephone (N = 6).

General questions for AD-diagnosed respondents included how their life and/or identity had changed since diagnosis; how they made sense of their condition; their opinions regarding the general public's awareness of their condition; and what they perceived as their role in informing research and care. Questions for the Association staff included job description and duties; the objectives of both the organisation and their department; obstacles to these aims; how they defined AD; what they saw as the role of individuals with AD within the Association; what was being done, on either an individual or organisational level, to encourage the visibility of diagnosed spokespeople, and existing barriers thereto.

Internal, external and historical obstacles to incorporating spokespersons

Respondents with AD highlighted a resounding willingness to become more visible in the dialogue surrounding dementia, the role they could play in this effort, and the obstacles they perceived to such endeavours. They noted that voicing their concerns satisfied a need to 'do something' during a time of heightened uncertainty:

> To come together like we have here today and say, 'Let's talk about what's happening and what we can do about it'. It's not enough to just curse the darkness. We need to get some light on the subject (83 year-old man).

> If you don't get out there and make yourself known and heard . . . I need to have the knowledge that I'm doing what I can . . . and that helps . . . If you put yourself out there and identify who you are, what your problem is . . . (86-year-old man).

Unfortunately, they cited a variety of barriers preventing them from 'being heard', including the fact that the nature of the condition with which they had been diagnosed potentially obfuscated (first socially and eventually personally) their ability to advocate in a confident and compelling manner. This understanding included an awareness[3] of the shame associated with AD. Most importantly, despite these hesitations respondents resisted taking on AD and the 'deficiency perspective' (Booth and Booth 1999) surrounding it as a master status, and were eager to inform the movement in their name.

Respondents from the Association unanimously stressed the importance of incorporating perspectives of people with dementia into planning care, services and policies aimed at them:

> There's a real consciousness in the Alzheimer's Association . . . to engage people [with AD] and involve them (Interim President, National Office).

> [There] is a slowly growing voice [of people with AD] that's invited [to participate]. We want their voice as part of the . . . we want to include them in the association (Associate Executive Director, Southwest).

There were, however, various competing organisational needs conflicting with the stated objective. Some of these dynamics were within the Association itself and others were external factors similar to those confronting many voluntary organisations. The history and nature of the disease itself further prevented the realisation of this goal. The benefits and barriers to making space for the voice of people with AD will be discussed from the perspective of the representatives employed at the SMO serving them.

Association respondents were personally motivated in the struggle to help people with Alzheimer's and their families as most had a relative who had lived with AD. The staff highlighted the importance of including people with memory loss in the realm of research, policy-making and service delivery. Most centrally, they spoke of the benefit of putting a 'face' on the Association itself and suggested the most effective way to do so was by encouraging spokespersons from within the ranks of those living with memory loss:

> [T]here are people who . . . don't want people to know but there are just as many people who . . . don't mind sharing their stories to get the word out. [W]hen you're more visible . . . people become more vocal about demanding better care, . . . more money for research, . . . [and] making sure that the families and friends that they know get the care (Development and Communications, East Coast).

> We will . . . somehow . . . change the face of Alzheimer's disease to show these people who are able to speak for themselves, who are healthy, who work out everyday, who take care of their dogs, and who work on their computers (Executive Director, Northwest).

Although the Association's interest in the role people with the disease could have in increasing public knowledge of the condition, and subsequently their organisation, is possibly a form of co-optation, noteworthy efforts are being undertaken.

Many chapters were encouraging people with AD to 'plead their cause' by recruiting advocates from Association-sponsored support groups. Facilitators of these groups are ostensibly able to hand-select effective lobbyists. Since the (biomedical) knowledges and practices informing the Association's activities and official policy positions are often at odds with the perspectives of individuals with AD, however, these efforts conceivably aid the Association in procuring more attention and funding; 'putting a face' is also a strategic manoeuvre. Despite ardent intentions, there are a number of factors that complicate efforts to incorporate the perspectives of people with AD, including internal dynamics of the Association, external factors and overarching features.

Internal dynamics

On 10th April 1980, representatives from five family support groups and staff from the National Institutes of Health and the National Institute on

Aging cited two primary objectives in forming the Alzheimer's Disease and Related Disorders Association, Inc. (ADRDA): increasing public awareness and the search for a cure. By 1988, dropping the 'and Related Disorders' solidified a constituency and clearly demarcated the organisational objectives of the Alzheimer's Association. This single-disease orientation is still evident today:

> The Alzheimer's Association, a national network of chapters, is the largest national voluntary health organization dedicated to advancing Alzheimer's research and helping those affected by the disease. The Association ranks as the top private funder of research into the causes, treatments, and prevention of Alzheimer's disease. The Association also provides education and support for people diagnosed with the condition, their families, and caregivers.

> In addition, advocacy is a major component of the Alzheimer's Association mission to achieve a world without Alzheimer's disease. We have emerged as an authority on the issues that affect people with Alzheimer's disease and their families, serving as a voice for them in the capitals of every state, hundreds of US congressional offices, and even the White House (Alzheimer's Association 2004a).

Since the historical foundation of the Association was primarily based on input from professionals trying to eradicate the condition and on families trying to cope with the stress and burden associated with what was at the time considered the 'disease of caregivers', vast contributions have been made in both areas. Diagnostic efficacy has greatly improved, allowing for much earlier diagnoses, and there are now four FDA-approved medications thought to slow decline in the early to moderate stages[4]. Significant work aimed at family support within the social and behavioural sciences[5] has translated the perspectives of care-partners into public policy and the Association's efforts. The founding ideals focusing on bench research and family support have also meant that people with the disease, and their perspectives, were often overlooked. Thus, factors within the Association preventing the incorporation of people with AD include organisational habits, organisational survival and organisational structure.

Organisational habits
The role of cutting-edge scientific discoveries, new pharmaceutical treatments, a population that is ageing, a variegated group of diagnosed individuals, and the relatively new phenomenon of including the perspectives of people with dementia, all contribute to the dynamic environment embedding AD. Combined with scientific and family-support underpinnings, respondents suggest that these dynamics obstruct the incorporation of diagnosed people into the debate even within the Association itself:

The primary barrier [to incorporating people with AD as spokespersons] may simply be working through habits (Public Policy, Midwest).

We're like all organizations in that we've been doing things in a certain way and it's hard to change. And the people that we serve [now] are the people with the disease . . . that's changed since I've been with the Association, but it's been emerging over the last decade (Interim President, National Office).

Organisational habits that aimed to find respite for families were consistent with the curative focus of founding scientists. Unfortunately, both of these factors impede the inclusion of people with AD regardless of the avowed aims. The primary organisational habit is a biomedical focus, including the allocation of over $150 million to predominantly bench science since 1982 (Alzheimer's Association 2004b).

Organisational survival

As a non-profit-making agency, the Association relies heavily on private donations. This impacts on at least two realms relevant to the inclusion of the diagnosed perspective: the public image that is to be portrayed and how money should be allocated. As a voluntary organisation, the Association does marketing to increase awareness of their services and certain things sell better than others. Unfortunately, the Association has not always encouraged favourable portrayals of people with the condition.

As with childhood conditions (Stockdale 1999), depictions of 'pathetic' victims are essential tools for fund-raising, despite the fact that this is no longer the (only) picture to portray. Along with epidemic projections, notions of a complete annihilation of self have historically served the Association well in their efforts to garner sympathisers (*i.e.* employing fear to advance resources). Portraying apocalyptic demography (Robertson 1990) and notions of scientific progress as combat is a mechanism necessary to unify members and help elicit support under the common goal of disease eradication. The respondents highlighted this tension:

It creates an interesting dilemma for us. The more you emphasize that people have rich lives and should have and should play more of a role . . . but think about the flip side of that: 'Oh, Alzheimer's isn't so bad. Look at all the creativity, and look at how wonderful . . .' . . . it's fraught with complications. How do you reconcile with the need to tell people that this disease is awful, and that we should get rid of it. That it isn't a good thing to live with this disease. So you're constantly juggling . . . if you allow one picture to dominate, you get a distorted view (Interim President, National Office).

What we have to do is make sure we're protecting human rights at the same time we're letting the world know how awful and ugly and destructive the disease is. Separating the human, the person, from the disease is a trick because you need the person to exhibit the disease (Public Policy, Washington, DC).

The contradiction herein is one facing many non-profit-making organisations serving constituencies deemed 'vulnerable'.

Thus, the Association must 'orchestrate' the need for public awareness and education because its members and staff believe, based on medico-scientific 'fact', that a disease exists which demands attention (Gubrium 1986). Demographically, financially, socially and personally, the problem is portrayed as devastating and warranting resources matching its prevalence, thus echoing the Association's ethos and scientific investigations behind it. The complicated and mysterious nature of the disease continues to aid the Association in its efforts to excite adequate monetary and human investments in the cause, as the website depicts:

Hope, formerly nonexistent, is growing. Scientists are slowly solving the disease's mysteries . . . Within five years treatments could be available to delay or prevent the disease (Alzheimer's Association 2004c).

Reminiscent of the Nixon era's War on Cancer, predictions of cutting-edge breakthroughs combined with catastrophic projections are effective efforts to create hype for investment (Stockdale 1999). These representations, however, also have unrecognised consequences for people with AD that fragment the face of the social movement in irrefutable ways.

Regarding resource allocation, most funding comes from people in the community with personal experiences of the condition. Thus, respondents noted that funds tend to be earmarked:

Most people when they're asked what we should be doing say, 'You should be doing more research'. That's where the general population thinks we should be investing all of our time. The caregivers they couldn't care less about. The people that care about the caregivers and those issues are the families that are dealing with it [who are the primary contributors] (Development and Communications, East Coast).

Therefore, discrepancies between where patrons prefer monies go and where the general public, and arguably the Association, thinks they should go (*i.e.* programmes vs. advertising) are likely.

The Association staff perceive a lack of adequate funding to devise and implement new objectives[6]. Many chapters do not seek foundation funding and few, if any, obtain government support. Respondents propose that financial constraints result in encouraging those services that reach the most people, are the most cost-effective, and are fundable:

There's the whole utilitarian thing of do I try to help the most people a little or a few people a lot? I try to help a lot of people at least a little and you hope it helps some of them a lot, but you at least go for the broad effect (Public Policy, Washington, DC).

An organisation historically addressing the needs of families particularly well requires substantial reorganisation first to identify and then to meet the requirements of this new clientele. Accordingly, the Association would have to begin by answering the question of who their client was and then either redirect or expand their efforts. Thus, individualised services are costly and beneficial to fewer people than standard caregiver-based or group programmes.

Organisational structure

Another internal obstacle to incorporating the voice of people with AD is the decentralised structure of the Association. There are currently 167 free-standing chapters, with representation in all 50 states[7]. Decisions directly relevant to the population each chapter serves are made at a local level. Although the Association has an impressive web presence, the devolution of services suggests little unifying chapters more broadly. Some respondents implied that this might create a lack of cohesion on the issue of personal advocacy:

It [incorporating people with AD] is probably more prevalent in the metropolitan chapter areas . . . It's only us because we have a longstanding history with early stage, but in the other offices [it is] not so much. I think that's probably pretty typical. There are chapters that don't even have support groups for people with the condition (Executive Director, Northwest).

Currently, there is no official Association policy on such endeavours, therefore some chapters are pioneers in the efforts to incorporate people with AD and others simply lack the resources, savvy or impetus for any such initiatives. The focus of local chapters on individual communities potentially obfuscates the unification of all Association staff on the larger social justices upon which the movement is based.

External factors

The internal dynamics identified delineate conflicting ideologies within the Association, which are exacerbated by the external factors confronting them, including public perceptions of ageing and AD, the role of science/medicine and client characteristics.

Public perceptions

Many depictions of Alzheimer's disease are skewed, if not outright pejorative, as a general cynicism pervades the discourse on topics of ageing and AD. Respondents attributed much of the struggle over including voice to larger issues of ageism:

> I fear that because of a level of ageism in public life and in private life that what gets public officials' attention more is the person who is still in his or her working years. It makes it all the more, 'My, god! This could be me' (Public Policy Director, Midwest).

> I think that probably the bigger problem is ageism and that age is still discounted to some extent. You know, old people get sick and they die (Education/Support Group Manger, East Coast).

As an organisation in the voluntary sector, various dilemmas regarding appeals for support are encountered. Considering demand-side client characteristics (Billis and Glennerster 1998), the Association serves people suffering from both personal and societal disadvantages. Accordingly, personal disadvantage occurs when ability to communicate is deemed impaired. As people with AD allegedly required others to act on their behalf, professionals and families of people with AD historically served as interpreters of their perspectives. Groups neglected within society experience a social disadvantage generated by the conflation of ageing and disease or other forms of discrimination. The social death upon which these assumptions are based marginalises people with AD, thus silencing their agenda.

Respondents also noted that the general public holds a number of misconceptions about the condition and people with it. First, many people believe that AD is an old person's disease, which despite statistical acuity risks minimising the experiences of people so diagnosed. In fact, although the vast majority of people are over 65 years of age, up to 10 per cent of AD cases are people diagnosed in their forties and fiftes with early-onset AD (Mattson 1998). Many people also consider it normal to have some memory loss as people age and, hence, risk conflating ageing and disease (Beard and Estes 2002). Another common portrayal is that of a sudden onset and a catastrophic outcome. In reality, AD is a gradual process with significant variation in the ensuing 8–20 years people can live with the condition.

Respondents suggested that a general paternalism surrounds the treatment of people with AD. In particular, family members might not want their loved ones to be spokespeople so as to prevent them from being publicly humiliated:

> There are so many families and individuals where if you go to them and say, 'We'd like you to be a spokesperson', they won't because of not wanting to deal with the public perception and the stigma or just the unwelcome encouraging words (Public Policy, Washington, DC).

Further, there is a general sense among many families, service providers and Association staff that people with AD (necessarily) require protection.

Poignantly, the type of person respondents thought would be most persuasive as a spokesperson poses serious dilemmas. Association staff envisaged someone famous, young and late-stage. They collectively noted a need for a spokesperson of celebrity status[8], such as Christopher Reeves or Michael J. Fox. Accordingly, younger people with AD (early-onset) are more tragic and resonate more powerfully with politicians, particularly in the later stages:

> The challenge is that people in the very early stages look very normal, and sometimes there's a bit of disconnect. They say, 'Well gee, he doesn't look so bad. That person is functioning pretty well'. Some of the most effective testimony has been with a person present who is actually fairly far advanced in the disease, but who is themselves not old . . . when they look at a 58-year-old fighter pilot who's owned his own business and is very handsome and looks much like the legislator sitting there across from him, there's some connection. And when they see that guy sitting there muted by Alzheimer's disease, that's pretty powerful. When your 85-year-old grandmother is going senile [people think], 'Well, she's just old and that's what happens'. So, I don't think there is the same sense of urgency as when you look at somebody who's 65 and go, 'Oh my god!' (Director of Development and Communications, East Coast).

The inherent contradiction herein is that cases of early-onset AD are extremely rare and have a far more rapid progression, thus complicating their ability to serve as spokespeople. Respondents highlighted preclinical cases of AD, including genetic predisposition and the emergence of Mild Cognitive Impairment (MCI), as far more compelling spokespeople yet full of ethical quandaries surrounding debates on diagnostic efficacy, genetic testing and the Human Genome Project. Therefore, although both the Association and the movement benefit from the nosological expansion of classification systems (Hedgecoe 2003) it engenders medical and public uncertainty and exacerbates ethical dilemmas.

The role of science/medicine
In theory and in practice, both science and medicine have played profound roles in the Alzheimer's movement and its leading SMO. Physicians in clinical practice, however, constitute a (potential) factor inhibiting the Association from employing the voices of people with AD. Importantly, there is considerable scientific controversy surrounding a unified definition of dementia and debates regarding whether or not AD is qualitatively different from normal ageing persist[9]. Since Alzheimer's cannot be definitively determined pre-mortem, the accuracy of diagnostic procedures varies (McAllister and Powers 1994). As people age, it is even more difficult to discern 'pure' cases of AD since few are without co-morbidities. For those who are diagnosed,

there are no magic bullets to cure AD and there are no 'survivors' as there are with other health social movements, which compounds the disadvantage of people with AD and amplifies obstacles to self-advocacy.

All of these issues confound the diagnostic process in clinical practice. Specifically, Association respondents noted a breakdown of education regarding the Association's services and AD more broadly on behalf of doctors:

> The biggest barrier [to including people with AD] I see is lack of knowledge on the part of physicians, which also leads to them not identifying it [AD] (Public Policy Director, Southwest).

> In every training I have done in the last 11 years the issue of physicians has come up: they don't know enough, they don't diagnose, they don't treat, they don't refer . . . the only thing that is going to change physician behavior is equipping the consumer to get more out of that physician visit (State Policy and Advocacy Program, Washington, DC).

Despite earlier diagnoses, when people *can* talk about their condition freely, doctors are allegedly not channelling people to the Association quickly enough, if at all. In this way, Association staff viewed doctors as the linchpin to solving some of their internal barriers:

> You ask people where do they get their information and they say their physician . . . You have to create a culture [of referral] within the physician community. To try to educate physicians [is] really tough because how do you get them, and, why should they care what the Alzheimer's Association says? (Interim President, National Office).

> I think getting physicians to refer people to us. We have to get that. I mean if our goal is to get to people early and support them through the journey, we have to partner with physicians, or physicians have to partner with us. I think that is the huge barrier (Executive Director, Northwest).

Given the Association's biomedical tenets, this discrepancy between diagnosing and referring people being attributed to a lack of knowledge on behalf of the doctors 'conveniently recreates the authoritative position' (Stockdale 1999) of biomedical *solutions* as opposed to their being part of the cause. Efforts to educate consumers (people with AD and their families) arguably have the same effect of assigning blame because of lack of information.

Client characteristics

There are also characteristics specific to the clientele that potentially prevent the perspectives of people with AD. First, respondents spoke of a cohort effect where seniors are less comfortable speaking about personal experiences to their doctors:

> I think there's the beginning of a cohort effect, where you've got people who are more willing to talk about this. Older generations may be a little more shy about it, even if they could do it (Interim President, National Office).

> The cohort of people who are that age [80s] are kind of shy about this advocacy business. Generationally, you just didn't speak about these things (Public Policy, Washington, DC).

Although such characteristics currently raise serious problems, respondents were confident that times would change with the ageing of the baby-boomers:

> [C]learly with the boomers aging our way of looking at aging is changing and is going to continue to change. [They] don't buy that they have to be decrepit and are less likely to say, 'Ah, that's just aging' and accept it. I think that the boomers are more likely to ask their . . . physicians questions and to seek alternative medicines if the medicine doesn't help them . . . they'll fight (Associate Executive Director, Southwest).

> The baby boomers are saying, 'We're not going to put up with this. We are going to question our doctor, we're going to figure out what's wrong, and we are going to come out in the open' (Education/Support Group Manger, East Coast).

The second client characteristic confounding the incorporation of their perspectives is the sheer variability between people who have AD. Respondents noted this conflict:

> [If] [e]very case of Alzheimer's is a new case of Alzheimer's, [then] . . . take that new case of Alzheimer's to a family, which all families are different with their own dynamics, so there's another new situation and so I don't think there's any [one] thing . . . a little bit of extra finances would help but the financial is not the, it's just one of many, many burdens involved with this (Chapter CEO, East Coast).

> Because it varies from person to person and it has so many different effects on everybody . . . there are so many different layers. It's hard to pinpoint one thing for them to look after [i.e. advocate] when it just varies so much (Communications Coordinator, Midwest).

Differences including age, education, ethnicity, class, gender, degree of other impairments and stage of the condition, threaten to preclude cohesion, a group identity and a unified public image.

Historical milieu: an overarching obstacle

Another crucial factor related to conveying the perspectives of people with AD is the pathology of the disease itself, which exacerbates both internal and external barriers. The dilemmas the Association has encountered in trying to change its image and orientations from a focus on families to those with the condition have important ramifications. Health social movements often work for the benefit of carers, whose activism is often crucial to building SMOs. Compared with diseases that do not affect memory, and combined with late-stage diagnoses, the Alzheimer's movement was initially required to organise around families. Now that people with AD are diagnosed far earlier in the disease trajectory, however, notions of families as the real victims are problematic. Unfortunately, the site of pathology leads many to make assumptions of incompetence due to western perceptions of brain functioning as defining humanness. The aetiology itself also confounds the situation since traditional 'deficiency perspectives' (Booth and Booth 1999) view symptomatic forgetfulness as an impediment to communication. This connection between personhood and mind has created a 'hypercognitive society' (Post 1995), whereby diseases of the brain threaten the very essence of a person's 'being' in the world. Similar to childhood conditions organised around proxy advocates, a history of family advocacy is particularly difficult to combat even when articulate people with the condition emerge (Stockdale 1999). Despite the increasing availability of people with AD to advocate, the social construction of AD is resistant to debunking suppositions of ineptness.

Further, learning to incorporate a new constituency is laborious, and possibly less effective for purposes of attaining support. The efforts devoted to brand a personal face for AD so clearly advocated for by Association staff are hindered by historical factors. The (past) social construction of the disease as a condition where people were often diagnosed without any awareness of their situation led to many of the (present) views that people with AD cannot advocate for themselves. The current availability of people in the earliest stages renders a large group of people who are high-functioning and will live far longer with the condition. As a result of this dynamic, the Association has yet to reach equilibrium with the diagnostic processes allowing for, if not demanding, such incorporation. Although related to the external factors of both public perception and the role of science/medicine, these views are largely the result of the protracted translation of science to the public. Efforts to implement spokespersons from a group of people with a progressive degenerative disease pose dilemmas for the Association:

> To use an awful term, when you're 'branding', my hunch is you can't brand as easily and as quickly for someone who is going to go away. So, you do it but you have to know that you can't do it as much as you could with the caregiver or with the public personality . . . It probably takes a lot

of work to cultivate someone into being an effective spokesperson and you know that there is a window of time. So, to be perfectly cold and blunt about it . . . you know their day will come sooner, when they can't – no matter what their drive, they physically and cognitively won't be able to anymore (Public Policy, Washington, DC).

Accordingly, planning speaking engagements would be difficult since it is unpredictable how a person might be feeling. Therefore, advocates who have a shorter 'window of time' are seen as less effective than unimpaired care-partners or celebrities. Thus, unlike disease-based movements where progression or signifying characteristics does not result in (cognitive) impediments to advocacy efforts, the intersection of disease pathology and the Association's mobilisation strategies are critical. The historical and social constructions of AD further confound the quandary of internal and external barriers to implementing spokespersons.

Overall, elements both internal and external to the Association as well as the environment embedding the condition must be acknowledged. The disparities between what the Association personally and publicly wants and what is organisationally feasible are significant. These dynamics are important for other health social movements serving similarly disadvantaged groups to take into account. We may begin to find the (attempted) utilisation of spokespersons earlier in the course of illness whose conditions are less visibly noticeable and/or are more receptive to pharmaceutical treatments than in the past.

Conclusions: despite best intentions

The Alzheimer's disease movement is credited for encouraging the emergence of AD as a social problem that recast the disease from a relatively rare phenomenon to the fourth or fifth leading cause of death in the United States in just one decade (Fox 1989). The mobilisation of resources that advanced and organised the AD movement occurred within a context of structural and socio-psychological conditions that contributed to the creation of a movement necessary to cultivate the presentation of AD as a significant problem. By exploring how the AD movement responds to and impacts on the voice of AD-diagnosed people, future studies can begin to bridge micro-experiences and larger structural forces by examining how health social movement organisations influence illness experiences, and vice versa. The mechanisms of transmission, methods of diagnosis, sites of pathology, course of progression, management and affected populations all influence the groups organising around them.

Although biomedical constructions of AD serve as a unifying force within the Association, the increased sophistication of diagnostic technologies yielding vast numbers of people far earlier in the disease process has not had the anticipated effect of bringing to the forefront personal accounts of the condition. This is arguably because the Association, and the movement upon which it is based, elevates certain goals (*e.g.* a cure) precluding others (*e.g.* quality of life). As with other single-agenda organisations (Stockdale 1999), the Association neglects potentially competing concerns; the biomedical ethos impedes an understanding of the many ways people live with and experience the disease. Such rival ideologies engender conundrums for serving people with AD and their loved ones.

While external funding allows the provision of more, often badly needed, services, monies can exert strong pressures on SMOs to organise in ways consistent with funding sources. This may result in an organisational focus primarily on providing more programmes and sponsoring more research at the expense of policy initiatives and more dynamic changes. The situation is confounded by the fact that the majority of financial resources come from individual donors aiming for increased and improved services directed at the people with AD and their loved ones.

Despite the availability and willingness of people with AD to speak about their experiences, both they and Association staff perceive various barriers to this integration. On an organisational level, organisational routines, the pursuit of funding, and a decentralised organisational structure prevent the incorporation of people with the disease. Regardless of intentions, there nonetheless exist inherent biases within the Association in favour of biomedical aims and caregivers as the primary clients. Beyond the Association, external factors including public perceptions, the role of science/medicine and client characteristics obstruct these intentions. An overarching obstacle encumbering the Association's ability to incorporate these perspectives is the disease pathology itself. Both the social construction of AD historically and western links between personhood and brain functioning encourage organisational habits of paternalism despite compelling, if recent, data suggesting otherwise. More first-person accounts of AD should continue to reverse the trend suggesting people with Alzheimer's cannot effectively organise and campaign.

The perspectives of people with AD have yet to be fully integrated into the philosophy of the Association, arguably as a result of the social death experienced upon diagnosis. Despite the fact that encouraging more people with AD to speak publicly can benefit the Association's efforts, the incorporation of personal spokespersons for the AD movement suffers the same biomedical and caregiver biases as does so much of Alzheimer's research and practice. Although diagnostic advances aid the Association by offering access to people in earlier stages of the disease, the biomedical, social, political and economic forces converging continue to generate significant obstacles. Given the perception that people with AD are incompetent as advocates, barriers may relate to biomedical foci of the organisation itself that do not address such misconceptions about people living with Alzheimer's. Attempts to bridge the gap between the biomedical/caregiver focus and the perspectives of those with AD will prove essential.

The Association's efforts have resulted in the elevation of certain agendas, presumably for the sake of more emancipatory efforts such as combating the conflation of ageing and disease or Alzheimer's and social death. Such diffusion risks transforming a social movement into an interest group working for moderate reform from within existing sociopolitical processes and structures. If the Association appears to be a formal, professional organisation working for reform through conventional methods, then it is not surprising that obstacles to including people with AD are so pervasive.

These data highlight not only the difficulty in incorporating narratives of people with AD into biomedical structures and the social movements based on them, but also of other populations, such as children and those with mental illnesses or learning disabilities, whose voices have been similarly silenced. Despite the considerable potential to recruit advocates from support groups to lobby as members of the social movement, that so few chapters currently do so is probably a result of the contradictions within the Association. Other health social movements where support groups are not sponsored by SMOs may prove more fruitful in incorporating the perspective of their constituencies. At present, the recent 'advances' made regarding dispensing the perspectives of people with AD only exacerbate the Association's already severe schism between achieving biomedical and client objectives.

Acknowledgements

The author would like to thank all the individuals who took the time to voice their opinions and speak about their experiences. This project could not have been done otherwise. Thank you as well to Adam Z. Bard, for your invaluable input, and Dale Rose, for your encouragement to take this further. The comments from the editors and two anonymous reviewers also significantly improved this manuscript.

Notes

1 It is not that the disability or mental health movements has not proposed other models, namely social, to combat the medical model but the activists from both of these movements have been less resistant to modern medical approaches than members of AIDS or breast cancer movements. Consequently, relationships between social movements and medicine vary significantly.

2 The Dementia Advocacy and Support Network (DASN) International was founded as an on-line support group in 2000 and has since expanded to a non-profit-making organisation comprising approximately 200 members. The endeavours being pursued to incorporate the perspectives of people with dementia (PWiDs) speak to the desires and unmet needs of PWiDs to be included in the debates surrounding dementia.

3 Space constraints make it implausible to discuss debates surrounding the subject of awareness/insight more generally. Focus group respondents, by definition of support group participation, were not in denial. The interviewees, however, did

not have the same exclusion criteria. Nonetheless, the researcher is confident none of these respondents were in denial at the time they were involved in this study.

4   The US Food and Drug Administration (FDA) has approved two classes of drugs to treat cognitive symptoms of Alzheimer's disease. The first Alzheimer medications to be approved were cholinesterase inhibitors, three of which are commonly prescribed. The second class are known as N-methyl-D-aspartate (NMDA) receptor antagonists and the only Alzheimer drug of this type was made available in the United States in October 2003 (Alzheimer's Association, 2004:b). *Treatments for Alzheimer's Disease.* Retrieved 31/01/2004 from http://www.alz.org/AboutAD/Treatment/Standard.htm).

5   For example, Aneshensel *et al.* 1995, Gordon *et al.* 1996, Lawton *et al.* 1991, Noonan and Tennstedt 1997, Zarit *et al.* 1998.

6   This is possibly in part due to the emerging need to expand services to address the needs of people with AD.

7   This number has steadily decreased since 1993, when there were 221 chapters (Alzheimer's Association (2004). *About Us: Timeline.* Retrieved 31/01/2004 from http://www.alz.org/AboutUs/History/overview.htm).

8   Since 1998, David Hyde Pierce (famous sitcom actor) has done extensive advocacy for the Association. His perspectives, however, are not first-hand but as a public official aiming to garner support. Princess Yasmin Aga Khan, daughter of the late Rita Hayworth, also currently serves on the Association's Board of Directors.

9   For example, Beach 1987, Fox 1989, Herskovits 1995, Ming and Fernandez 2001.

References

Alzheimer's Association (2004) *About Us: Overview.* Retrieved 31/01/2004 from (A) http://www.alz.org/AboutUs/overview.htm

Alzheimer's Association (2004) *About Us: Timeline.* Retrieved 31/01/2004 from (B) http://www.alz.org/AboutAD/Treatment/Standard.htm

Alzheimer's Association (2004) *About Us: History.* Retrieved 31/01/2004 from (C) http://www.alz.org/AboutUs/History/overview.htm

Aneshensel, C.S., Pearlin, L.I., Mullan, J.T., Zarit, S.H. and Whitlatch, C.J. (1995) *Profiles in Caregiving: the Unexpected Career.* New York: Academic Press.

Beach, T.G. (1987) The history of Alzheimer's disease: three debates, *Journal of the History of Medicine and Allied Sciences,* 42, 327–49.

Beard, R.L. (2004) In their voices: identity preservation and experiences of Alzheimer's disease, *Journal of Ageing Studies,* 18, 4.

Beard, R.L. and Estes, C.L. (2002) Medicalization of Aging. *Macmillan Encyclopedia of Aging.* New York: Macmillan Press.

Billis, D. and Glennerster, H. (1998) Human services and the voluntary sector: towards a theory of comparative advantage, *Journal of Social Policy,* 27, 1, 79–98.

Bond, J. (1992) The medicalization of dementia, *Journal of Ageing Studies,* 6, 397–403.

Booth, T. and Booth, W. (1999) Parents together: action research and advocacy support for patients with learning difficulties, *Health and Social Care in the Community,* 7, 6, 464–74.

Braudy Harris, P. (2002) *The Person with Alzheimer's Disease: Pathways To Understanding the Experience.* Baltimore, MD: Johns Hopkins University Press.

Canguilhem, G. (1991) *On the Normal and the Pathological.* New York: Zone Books.

Cheston, R. and Bender, M. (1999) *Understanding Dementia: the Man with the Worried Eyes.* London: Jessica Kingsley Publishers.

Cohen, D. (1991) The subjective experience of Alzheimer's disease: the anatomy of an illness as perceived by patients and families, *American Journal of Alzheimer's Care and Related Disease and Research,* 6–11 May/June.

Corbin, J.M. and Strauss, A. (1998) *Basics of Qualitative Research: Techniques and Procedures for Developing Grounded Theory,* 2nd Edition, New York: Sage Publications.

Cottrell, V. and Schulz, R. (1993) The perspective of the patient with Alzheimer's disease: a neglected dimension of dementia research, *The Gerontologist,* 32, 205–11.

Cutler, N. (1986) Public response: The national politics of Alzheimer's disease. In Gilhooly, M., Zarit, S. and Birrens, J. (eds) *The Dementias: Policy and Management.* NJ: Prentice Hall.

Davis, R. (1989) *My Journey into Alzheimer's Disease.* Illinois: Tyndale House Publishers.

DeBaggio, T. (2002) *Losing my Mind: an Intimate Look at Life with Alzheimer's.* New York: The Free Press.

Dyer, J. (1996) *In a Tangled Wood.* Dallas: Southern Methodist University Press.

Epstein, S. (1996) *Impure Science: AIDS, Activism, and the Politics of Knowledge.* Berkeley: University of California Press.

Fox, P.F. (1989) From senility to Alzheimer's disease: the rise of the Alzheimer's disease movement, *The Millbank Quarterly,* 67, 1, 58–102.

Fox, P.F. and Muller, M.R. (2001) *Disease-based Social Movements and Health Policy Reform: Alzheimer Disease and Acquired Immune Deficiency Syndrome.* University of California, San Francisco: Institute for Health and Aging.

Friel-McGowin, D.F. (1993) *Living in the Labyrinth: a Personal Journey through the Maze of Alzheimer's.* New York: Dell Publishing.

Glaser, B.G. and Strauss, A.L. (1966) *Awareness of Dying.* London: Weidenfeld and Nicholson.

Glaser, B. and Strauss, A. (1967) *Discovery of Grounded Theory: Strategies for Qualitative Research.* Chicago: Aldine de Gruyter.

Goldsmith, M. (1996) *Hearing the Voice of People with Dementia: Opportunities and Obstacles.* London: Jessica Kingsley Publishers.

Golomb, J., Kluger, A., Garrard, P. and Ferris, S. (2001) *Clinican's Manual on Mild Cognitive Impairment.* London: Science Press.

Gordon, S., Benner, P. and Noddings, N. (1996) *Caregiving: Readings in Knowledge, Practice, Ethics, and Politics.* Philadelphia: University of Pennsylvania Press.

Gubrium, J. (1986) *Oldtimers and Alzheimer's: the Descriptive Organization of Senility.* Greenwich, CT: JAI Press.

Gubrium, J. (1987) Structuring and destructuring the course of illness: the Alzheimer's disease experience, *Sociology of Health and Illness,* 9, 1–24.

Hedgecoe, A.M. (2003) Expansion and uncertainty: cystic fibrosis, classification and genetics, *Sociology of Health and Illness,* 25, 1, 50–70.

Henderson, C. (1998) *Partial View: an Alzheimer's Journal.* Dallas: Southern Methodist University Press.

Herskovits, E. (1995) Struggling over subjectivity: debates about the 'Self' and Alzheimer's disease, *Medical Anthropology Quarterly,* 9, 2, 146–64.

Kastenbaum, R.J. (1969) Psychological death. In Pearson, L. (ed.) *Death and Dying*, OH: Case Western Reserve University Press.

Kitwood, T. and Bredin, K. (1992) Towards a theory of dementia care: personhood and well-being, *Ageing & Society*, 12, 269–87.

Klawiter, M. (1999) Racing for the cure, walking women, and toxic touring: mapping cultures of action within the Bay Area terrain of breast cancer, *Social Problems*, 46, 1, 104–26.

Kramer, L. (1989) *Reports from the Holocaust.* New York: St. Martin's Press.

Lawton, M.P., Moss, M., Kleban, M., Glicksman, A. and Rovine, M. (1991) A two-factor model of caregiving appraisal and psychological well-being, *Journal of Gerontology: Psychological Sciences*, 46, 81–9.

McAllister, M.D. and Powers, R. (1994) Approaches to the treatment of dementing illness. In Emery, V.O. and Oxman, T.E. (eds) *Dementia: Presentations, Differential Diagnosis, and Nosology.* Baltimore, MD: The Johns Hopkins University Press.

Mattson, M.P. (1998) Experimental models of Alzheimer's disease, *Science and Medicine*, March/April, 16–25.

Ming, C. and Fernandez, H. (2001) Alzheimer movement re-examined 25 years later: Is it a 'disease' or a senile condition in medical nature? *Frontiers in Bioscience*, 6, e30–40.

Noonan, A.E. and Tennstedt, S. (1997) Meaning in caregiving and its contribution to caregiver well-being, *The Gerontologist*, 37, 6, 785–94.

Post, S.G. (1995) *The Moral Challenge of Alzheimer's Disease.* Baltimore, MD: Johns Hopkins Press.

Robertson, A. (1990) The politics of Alzheimer's disease: a case study in apocalyptic demography, *International Journal of Health Services*, 20, 3, 429–42.

Rose, L. (1996) *Show me the way to go home.* San Francisco, CA: Elder Books.

Rucht, D. (1996) The impact of national contexts on social movement structures: a cross-movement and cross-national comparison. In McAdam, D. McCarthy, J. and Zald, M. (eds) *Comparative Perspectives on Social Movements.* New York: Cambridge University Press.

Sabat, S.R. (2001) *The Experience of Alzheimer's Disease: Life Through a Tangled Veil.* Oxford: Blackwell Publishers Ltd.

Sabat, S.R. and Harre, R. (1992) The construction and deconstruction of self in Alzheimer's disease, *Ageing & Society*, 12, 443–61.

Schutz, A. (1967) *The Phenomenology of the Social World.* Illinois: Northwestern University Press.

Stockdale, A. (1999) Waiting for the cure: mapping the social relations of human gene therapy research, *Sociology of Health and Illness*, 21, 5, 579–96.

Strauss, A. and Corbin, J. (1990) *Basics of Qualitative Research: Grounded Theory Procedures and Techniques.* London: Sage Publications.

Sudnow, D. (1967) *Passing On: the Social Organization of Dying.* Englewood Cliffs, NJ: Prentice Hall Inc.

Sweeting, H. and Gilhooly, M. (1997) Dementia and the phenomenon of social death, *Sociology of Health and Illness*, 19, 1, 93–117.

Wilkinson, H. (ed.) (2002) *The Perspectives of People with Dementia: Research Methods and Motivations.* London: Jessica Kingsley Publishers.

Zarit, S., Stephens, M., Townsend, A. and Greene, R. (1998) Stress reduction for family caregivers: effects of adult day care use, *Journal of Gerontology: Social Sciences*, 53B, 5, s267–77.

Chapter 8

Framing as a cultural resource in health social movements: funding activism and the breast cancer movement in the US 1990–1993
Emily S. Kolker

Introduction

In the past 20 years, health social movements (HSMs) in the US have undergone a significant shift. Previously, HSMs had focused primarily on problems of patient care, including access to healthcare and health services. More recently, HSMs have turned from 'the clinic' to 'the lab' and have begun to pursue federal research funding to determine the causes and cures for specific diseases (Brown *et al.* 2002, Epstein 1996) and the attendant public recognition of such diseases. Federal-level funding activism has required HSMs to draw on both structural and cultural resources in order to be successful in their efforts. Structurally, HSMs draw on resources such as political opportunity structure, the organisation of other social movements, tactics, networks and institutional relationships. More recently, scholars have bypassed this resource mobilisation perspective and have turned their attention to the cultural elements and resources of social movements (Fine 1995, Guigni 1998, McAdam 1994, Swidler 1986, 1995, Williams 1995). In addition, because HSM funding activists must persuade the public that a disease is a matter of national concern, HSM activists must, in Mills's terms (1959), redefine disease from a personal trouble to a public issue. To do so, they draw upon important cultural resources. While the extant literature thoroughly chronicles how HSMs have drawn on structural resources, with a few exceptions (Epstein 1996, 1997, Klawiter 1999b), less attention has been paid to how they mobilise cultural resources to construct successful claims. Relying on the 'cultural turn' in social movement scholarship (Johnston and Klandermans 1995, McAdam 1994, Swidler 1986, Williams 1995), this study demonstrates how breast cancer funding activists used culturally resonant frames to persuade audiences and to redefine breast cancer from a private problem of individual women to a major public health problem worthy of increased federal funding.

The increase in federal funding for breast cancer in the US between 1990 and 1993 serves as an exemplar of HSM funding activism that made use of cultural resources, in the form of culturally resonant frames, to advocate for increased, disease-specific federal funding. The years 1990 to 1993 were selected because it was the period in which the largest gains in federal funding for breast cancer research took place, and they specifically represent what I term 'funding activism'[1]. During this short period, federal funding for breast cancer research was increased from \$89 million in fiscal year 1991 to \$430 million in fiscal year 1993, an increase of \$341 million (Love and Lindsey 1997). While most accounts of the breast cancer movement include the increase in research funding as a major accomplishment, or analyse the structural resources leading to this success (Weisman 2000), few have developed an understanding of the range of resources employed by activists. More specifically, only a handful of accounts examine how breast cancer activists drew on cultural resources to persuade their audiences (Klawiter 1999a, Klawiter 1999b, Taylor and Whittier 1995, Taylor and Van Willigen 1996). Using a social constructionist approach (Spector and Kitsuse 1977) to Congressional testimony and media accounts of breast cancer activism in the early 1990s, this chapter identifies and analyses the three central frames used by breast cancer activists in the early 1990s to define breast cancer as a major social problem in need of increased federal research funding[2].

Framing and health social movements

Building on Goffman's (1974) conceptualisation of frames, social movement scholars have emphasised the importance of the interpretive schema, or 'frame' (Snow et al. 1986) used for mobilising collective action. While much of this scholarship has been concerned with the instrumental question of how successful social movement frames have been in recruiting participants, more recent scholarship has asked questions about the expressive, or cultural, elements of movements and movement frames (Klawiter 1999b, Polletta 1997, Reese and Newcombe 2003, Wuthnow 1989). Such scholarship approaches framing as a verb, something that social movement actors 'do' or embody (Klawiter 1999b), and emphasises that social movements are involved in the business of signifying work, or producing meaning in the process of action (Snow and Benford 1992, Benford and Snow 2000, Tarrow 1992, Taylor and Whittier 1995, Williams and Benford 2000). From this perspective, the importance of framing lies in the way that frames, as meaning-constructing systems (Taylor and Whittier 1995), draw upon cultural ideologies to connect with and persuade audiences (Epstein 1997, Snow et al. 1986), not how they represent rational calculations of recruitment and movement strategies (Polletta 1997). This chapter emphasises how social movement actors utilise cultural ideologies in their framing activities to construct persuasive and culturally resonant frames and redefine social conditions. This analysis is therefore concerned with frames as a cultural resource employed by breast cancer activists for the instrumental purpose of attaining increased research funding, and redefining breast cancer as a public problem.

The frames and attendant claims used by activists to define breast cancer as a public problem had a high degree of cultural resonance with their audiences, a condition necessary for the success of a social movement (Epstein 1997, Johnston et al. 1994, Mirola 2003, Snow et al. 1986). This analysis expands the range of movement activities to include the public speech actions (Johnston 1995) of activists by examining the public performance of breast cancer activist discourse. Without question, this use of culturally resonant frames represented important instrumental resources for making demands of the government. The act of giving Congressional testimony and giving statements to the media, after all, is a highly instrumental activity. In recent years, sociologists have paid more attention to the role of rhetoric and discourse in the construction of social problems generally (Best 1987, Williams and Williams 1995) and, more specifically, in the speech acts of social movements (Benford and Snow 2000, Fine 1995, Johnston 1995, Taylor and Whittier 1995). In this chapter I analyse the rhetoric of activist frames to account for two distinct, but inter-related phenomena: the cultural resonance of activist frames with target audiences, and the redefinition of breast cancer from a private problem of individual women to a national public health problem.

Bringing breast cancer into the public eye

Though federal funding specifically for breast cancer research did not become a legitimate social problem until the early 1990s, it built on prior historical moments in the social construction of breast cancer in the public sphere. Before 1990, breast cancer had largely been defined as a problem of stigma, treatment screening and public health. In the 1970s, breast cancer began its journey into the public domain as well-known women in the US publicly shared their experiences of breast cancer, including Shirley Temple Black, Betty Ford and Happy Rockefeller (Altman 1996, Boehmer 2000, Weisman 2000). Prior to the publication of such high-profile stories, breast cancer was largely viewed as a private, and often shameful, experience of individual women, a topic better left in the past, and exclusively within close family and friendship networks (Leopold 1999, Taylor and Van Willigen 1996). Also beginning in the 1970s, and continuing throughout the 1980s, breast cancer treatment and detection became key focal points in the public discourse and politics of breast cancer. In particular, advocates challenged breast cancer treatment – radical Halsted mastectomy without informed consent (Lerner 2001, Montini 1996) – and sparked a legislative debate about the rights of patients to choose their course of treatment for breast cancer. Advocates lobbied at the state level and succeeded in establishing informed consent laws for breast cancer treatment in 16 states (Anglin 1997, Montini 1996). Simultaneously, breast cancer advocates also lobbied Congress to increase women's access to mammography (Weisman 2000). Lastly, in the mid-1980s, breast cancer was constructed by the media as an 'epidemic' (Lantz and Booth 1998), establishing a public perception that breast cancer was a major public health problem in the US.

The 1990s ushered in a new era of public claimsmaking about breast cancer that built on the media construction of a breast cancer epidemic. In

1990, an elite core of activists turned the focus of movement activity toward federal funding for breast cancer research, bypassing the dominant focus on advocacy for care and treatment[3]. Though policy efforts aimed at improving access to quality mammograms and treatment for breast cancer remained part of the larger breast cancer agenda, the most dramatic policymaking in the 1990s centred on increased governmental responsibility for breast cancer research (Weisman 2000). In shifting the focus of the movement in the early 1990s, activists drew attention away from the more clinical and individualistic problems of diagnosis, treatment and recovery and attempted to transform breast cancer from a private problem of individual women to a public health problem in need of a federal response.

Before 1990, fundraising efforts specific to breast cancer research were centred in private foundations, most notably the Susan G. Komen Breast Cancer Foundation, founder of the annual 'Race for the Cure' charity event. Therefore, by 1990 attention to increasing funding for breast cancer research was not in itself a radical idea, but activist demands that the federal government assume primary responsibility for such funding represented a significant shift in attribution for the problem of breast cancer. This relatively short period of funding activism defined governmental neglect of the disease, in the form of research funding, as the central problem associated with breast cancer. In this new context, breast cancer was constructed not as a problem of stigma or access to quality screening and treatment, but as a problem of insufficient scientific knowledge of the disease. In particular, this lack of scientific knowledge was linked back to the claim that government had not sufficiently prioritised research on breast cancer, furthering the epidemic of breast cancer through institutional neglect.

It is important to note that a cancer advocacy focus on governmental responsibility for funding scientific cancer research *in general* preceded the efforts of the breast cancer movement of the early 1990s. Beginning with the federally-mandated establishment of the National Cancer Institute in 1937, and continuing in the legislative efforts of cancer advocates in the passage of the National Cancer Act of 1971, cancer advocates historically made consistent public claims that government bore some responsibility for the state of insufficient funding and biomedical knowledge related to cancer (Rettig 1977, Ross 1987). Thus, breast cancer activists' efforts to increase federal funds for biomedical research in the early 1990s was not representative of a new venture in cancer advocacy. Instead, such activism represented a narrowing of pre-existing cancer policy to a funding and biomedical research agenda for a single form of cancer, in this case breast cancer (Klawiter 1999a).

Critical to the efforts of breast cancer funding activists was the 1990 formation of the National Breast Cancer Coalition (NBCC), the premier umbrella organisation under which hundreds of breast cancer organisations consolidated to create one body devoted to lobbying for breast cancer policies at the national level (Anglin 1997). Following the establishment of the

NBCC, lobbying increased around the first of the organisation's three priorities: federal funding for breast cancer research. In 1991, the NBCC launched its first efforts at increasing federal funds, including Congressional lobbying and a successful letter-writing campaign to President Bush, 'Do the Write Thing'. These initial efforts led to the appropriation of an additional $43 million for breast cancer research for fiscal year 1992, raising the research budget from $89 million to $132 million total (Love and Lindsey 1997). Encouraged by their initial success, activists lobbied Congress for an additional $300 million in research funds for fiscal year 1993. By the end of this period, breast cancer activists won their battle for increased federal funding for breast cancer research: by fiscal year 1993 federal breast cancer funding had increased from $89 million in fiscal year 1991 to $433 million in fiscal year 1993, a phenomenal political success.

The NBCC was represented most often by Dr. Susan Love, a well-known breast surgeon and author, and Fran Visco, President of the NBCC. In addition, individual breast cancer survivors, advocates, and occasional celebrities gave testimony before Congress and spoke to the media about the need for increased federal funding. The NBCC was the organisation most forceful in publicly defining breast cancer as a problem of governmental neglect. Thus, while other advocates bolstered the NBCC's requests for increased federal research funds, the NBCC took centre stage in redefining breast cancer as a public problem, and became the public face of breast cancer activism in the 1990s (Boehmer 2000).

The success of breast cancer funding activism was in part rooted in congressional activities and media coverage of the breast cancer movement at the time. Activists articulated their grievances to both politicians and the general public through claimsmaking in the form of congressional testimony, and through media coverage of movement activities. A Nexis database search for 'breast cancer' and 'funding' in national newspaper coverage for the years 1988–1992 yielded a dramatic picture of the amount of media attention given to federal funding. In 1988, only four articles appeared in national papers; by 1992 this number had risen to 103. As other scholars have noted, the success or failure of a social problem depends partly on the degree of public attention it can garner at any given time (Hilgartner and Bosk 1988). From 1990 to 1993, activists successfully claimed public space for breast cancer through their presence in Congress and extensive media coverage of their activities.

Claimsmaking for increased federal funding

In order to redefine breast cancer from a private problem of individual women to a major public health crisis in need of government intervention, activists relied on three core sets of culturally resonant frames in congressional testimony and media accounts of their activities: breast cancer as an epidemic, breast cancer as a problem of gender equity, and breast cancer as a threat to families. Interestingly, the set of frames used by breast cancer activists did not necessarily represent new definitions of the cancer problem in the context of the larger history of cancer legislation and politics in the US. Instead, activists appropriated previously employed frames and definitions of the broader problem of cancer in the 20th century to make their case for increased federal research monies. Consequently, what was new about the breast cancer movement in the early 1990s was the narrowing of the rhetoric of categorical disease research from cancer in general to breast cancer alone (Klawiter 1999a).

The epidemic of breast cancer

In their public speech acts, activists strove to redefine breast cancer as a major public health problem. They made the case for an unacceptable rate of breast cancer to justify their demands for increased funding. Activists were able to create this sense of urgency by drawing on the media's prior construction of a breast cancer 'epidemic' in the US (Lantz and Booth 1998). Activists argued publicly that women with breast cancer had too often been told that they would be fine – that they just needed to have a mastectomy, treatment, and return quietly to their old lives (*New York Times Magazine* 15 August 1993). These platitudes were understood by activists to reinforce the notion that breast cancer was a private problem of risk, diagnosis and treatment for individual women. With its emphasis on breast cancer awareness, diet, exercise and the importance of screening through mammograms, this personal responsibility model of breast cancer (Simpson 2000) was perceived by activists as placing blame for the disease on individual women. Dr. Love challenged these assumptions in a *JAMA* commentary titled What the Department of Defense Should Do with Its $210 Million:

> Why is breast cancer incidence increasing in the young and old? Some would have you believe that it is the fault of the woman herself (e.g., delayed pregnancy, too much dietary fat). But what of the societal causes? What about the carcinogens and hormones in the fat? (Love 1993: 2417).

Public statements like Dr. Love's redefined breast cancer as a potential epidemic of civilisation, environment and institutional neglect. Other advocates pointed out that if such high numbers of women were being struck with the disease, it must have been a problem of both the physical environment as well as institutional responses to the disease. While the demands for federal funds included other similar claims about the potential role of the environment in causing breast cancer, activists privileged the claim of neglectful institutional responses to an epidemic, and the necessity for increased funding to explore the avenues of potential causation. One such approach claimed that the government's funding priorities were misguided in a time of a national health crisis by focusing on defence spending at the cost of women's lives. Recognising that their demands coincided with the end of the Cold War, and that their success depended on the transfer of monies from the Defense Department for breast cancer research, activists argued for breast cancer funding as a type of peace dividend. The following testimony given by Dr. Love in a May 1992 hearing was followed by audience applause: 'New research money can be found. Not by stealing from other diseases . . . but by changing our priorities. We want less money for defending the country and more for defending our lives' (US Congress, Senate 4 May 1992: 18). NBCC President Fran Visco mirrored Dr. Love's testimony in an October 1992 hearing:

> Why can this country find $380 million for an obsolete project, but is unable to find $300 million to save women's lives? Why do we have to fight you so hard for this money? Why does this country continue to fund bombs and not the research that may save our lives and our daughters' lives? (US Congress, Senate 1 October 1992: 105).

Activist claims to the epidemic nature of breast cancer also included arguments about the national economic impact of the disease. Understanding that the allocation of federal monies for causes is distributed according to cost-benefit analyses, activists asserted that the disease annually cost the nation billions of dollars. In a July 1992 hearing, NBCC President Fran Visco stated:

> When you wanted to help the economy by creating jobs, you found a way to transfer millions for foreign aid to transportation. Recognize the impact of breast cancer on the economy. Breast cancer costs this country more than $8 billion [annually] in medical costs and lost productivity (US Congress, Senate 29 July 1992: 487).

Further, breast cancer activists recognised that the federal government was besieged by claims about conditions that affected specific populations, and further utilised the epidemic claim to assert that breast cancer affected all women, not just a proportion of 'high-risk' women (Weisman 2000). Because the notion of an epidemic had already been a focus of media coverage, activists' use of this claim resonated strongly with both Congressional and public audiences. Employing the epidemic claim, however, was not in itself enough to argue for government's responsibility for the disease. In addition, activists turned to the powerful master frame of gender equity to bolster their arguments.

Breast cancer as a problem of gender equity
Breast cancer activists simultaneously employed the master frame of gender equity (Weisman 2000, Williams and Williams 1995) with the epidemic claim. Specifically, the gender equity frame defined breast cancer as a problem of gender-based, institutional neglect. Activists adopted the gender equity

frame to define breast cancer as a public problem, mobilise supporters and account for the putative paucity of federal funds for breast cancer research. The use of an equity frame is common in social movements because it is easily recognisable to audiences (Snow and Benford 1992, Williams and Williams 1995), culturally potent (Williams and Benford 2000), and generally successful in the construction of social problems (Loseke 1999). Using this master frame, breast cancer activists elaborated on the gender-neutral frame of equity to include gender as a central organising feature of society (Taylor and Whittier 1995). The gender equity claim was easily mobilised by breast cancer activists as it had been used in prior women's movement and women's health movement activism in the US.

The collective action frame articulated by breast cancer activists in the early 1990s was the master frame of gender equity. Collective action frames are derivative of master frames in that they explain the cause of, and solution for, a problem (Williams and Williams 1995), but are issue-specific and produced through social movement activity (Snow and Benford 1992). In this case, activists used Congressional testimony and media coverage to frame breast cancer as a problem exacerbated by gender-based inequities in federal spending on research related to women's health. Activists forcefully contended that *because* breast cancer affected women, scientific knowledge about the disease had not received the public attention or the governmental funding that it deserved. Systematic, institutional neglect of women's health in the form of gender bias was claimed by activists to have contributed to the growing problem of breast cancer, and formed one of the 'grounds' (Best 1987) used to increase federal research funds. To make the gender-equity frame work, however, claimsmakers had to establish breast cancer as a disease of women, provide evidence for inequity in research funding, and create a viable bridge between activists and policymakers that would allow for a public connection to the problem of breast cancer. To make this first argument viable, activists consistently constructed breast cancer in public as a female disease despite the fact that men – though rarely in comparison to women – are also diagnosed and treated for the disease. In addition, activists identified as members of a collective and marginalised social group based on gender. At a 1992 hearing, Deanna Cooper, author of *1 in 9*, testified before Congress about her experience of breast cancer and the gendered dimensions of governmental neglect. She stated:

> While I have appeared before you as a quiet author expressing my personal fears and concerns, I want you to remember that I am a very angry woman, that my gender is dying, and that you and I could and must do much more (US Congress, Senate 4 May 1992: 31)[4].

Cooper reinforced the notion that breast cancer was a female disease, and made a strong claim of a threat to her gender as the result of discriminatory governmental neglect of breast cancer.

In addition to constructing breast cancer as a female disease, funding activists provided evidence of gender bias in federal research funding. The issue of federal funding for women's health-related research first caused a public ripple in 1990 with the release of a report investigating NIH practices conducted by the General Accounting Office that was instigated by the Congressional Women's Caucus. The GAO reported that the NIH was neglectful in following its own policy to include women in research, specifically in clinical trials. The investigation revealed two key findings about NIH practices related to research and women's health: that men continued to receive priority over women as research subjects in clinical trials, and that diseases associated with women received 15 per cent of the NIH's total $5.7 billion budget. At the time of the report, basic research on breast cancer received a total of $17 million from the NIH. This report led to the formation of a special NIH office on women's health issues, and prompted Dr. Bernadine Healy, the newly appointed Director of the NIH, to assure Congress that the NIH would develop a specific healthcare agenda for women. The GAO report, *New Leadership at the NIH*, and the political resource of the Congressional Women's Caucus provided evidence of a larger institutional context for gender bias that breast cancer activists used to further their demands for increased research funding.

Other claimsmakers made more coded reference to gender bias in federal research funding. For example, Ohio Congresswoman Mary Rose Oakar, whose sister had died of breast cancer, accused her colleagues of being inattentive to breast cancer while at the same time allocating resources to problems that affected men more than women:

Because of the Vietnam War, we lost 57,000 men and women. During that same period – we lost 330,000 women to breast cancer. So we're in a crisis, and yet there hasn't been the same zeal to do something about this issue as we see in other issues – and we do the right thing, I think, in other issues. Just to make a quick comparison, it was interesting to me that with respect to AIDS, we had $1.6 billion and, this year, the Budget Committee recommended 7,000,000 more dollars for AIDS research, which affects about one in every thousand individuals in this country- and I support that. However, we have been trying for some time to get an increase of about $25 million more for breast cancer research. In terms of pure research, we only spend about $19 million in that area. It has at times fallen on deaf ears (US Congress, Senate 16 May 1990).

The 'deaf ears' Oakar refers to clearly represent those of her colleagues, key policymakers who had the ability to allocate more money to breast cancer research, but had not done so in any significant way. Oakar also drew on a common tactic of claimsmakers for increased breast cancer funding – comparing the relative value of breast cancer to AIDS based on the amount of money each disease received from the government. Though

Oakar carefully acknowledged that dedicating funds to AIDS was the 'right thing' to do, her testimony implies that the government cared more about AIDS, coded by activists as a male disease, than they did about breast cancer[5].

Two years later, Fran Visco, President of the NBCC, echoed Oakar's claim of gender bias in federal spending for breast cancer:

> There are 2.8 million of us [breast cancer] survivors in this country today. This year has been touted as the year of the woman. In reality, it is just another year in which 46,000 of us will die of breast cancer. If the loss of life is not enough to spur Congress to find creative solutions, let us analyze this on a different basis. When the men in suits all but destroyed the savings and loan system in this country, the Nation's economic stability was threatened and this Congress responded with billions of dollars (Departments of Labor, Health and Human Services, and Education and Related Agencies Appropriation for Fiscal Year, 1993 28–30th July 1992: 487).

Both Oakar and Visco's testimony address the issue of gender bias, but in a far more coded manner than others who came to testify before Congress. Actress Lynda Carter, most famous for her portrayal of 'Wonderwoman', expressed anger at what she identified as a clear case of gender-based neglect of breast cancer as a woman's disease:

> I get angry sometimes that there's so many things that we could be doing in this country to combat breast cancer. I'm sorry to say this, but if this were an illness that were striking mostly men at the rate that it is striking women, I think that society's response would be much more swift and much more dramatic (US Congress, Senate 16 May 1990: 36)[6].

The claim of gender equity in federal research funding also surfaced in media stories, amplifying the claims made in the Congressional sphere. A *Cleveland Plain Dealer* article reported on the activist efforts of Nancy Chilcote, head of the Ohio branch of the NBCC, who strongly defined the problem of breast cancer as one of gender equity.

> 'I'm firmly convinced this is a gender problem', said Chilcote. 'If some part of a male sexual organ were being cut off at a rate of 1 in 9 in men, the world would stop rotating until we found a cure. Because it's a female disease, no one really cares' (*Plain Dealer*, 7 September 1993).

In an even stronger statement, Massachusetts State Senator Lois Pines blatantly attributed the state of breast cancer funding to gender discrimination and offered a clear solution:

We need to reverse the sexist allocation of Federal health care funding by greatly increasing the money that is spent on finding the cause as well as a cure for breast cancer (US Congress, Senate 4 May 1992: 25).

In contrast, Dr. Love, a well-known breast surgeon, author and a founding member of the NBCC, represented a more politic approach to breast cancer funding and gender equity. In a 1993 *LA Times* interview, Love defined the problem of gender equity in the federal allocation of research monies less as a conspiracy against women than a lack of personal connection with the disease. When asked to what extent such ignorance about breast cancer was related to it being a female disease, Love responded:

> I don't think the researchers are misogynists; I think if you're sitting there with a small pot of money, you will spend it on what you fear and if you're a middle-aged white male, it's more likely to go to heart disease than breast cancer . . . The reason we don't know more about breast cancer is that the people making the decisions didn't care enough about finding out those answers (*Los Angeles Times*, 5 December 1993).

Love's statement captures a problem that HSMs face in their attempts to increase federal funding for specific diseases: activist claims must resonate with multiple audiences, including the media, policymakers and the general public (Giugni 1998), to create a connection with their cause. The use of gender equity was a highly resonant frame that had proved successful in past political movements and had allowed activists to argue that breast cancer was not receiving adequate federal funding. In this case, however, the gender equity frame was employed at a time of increased political conservatism in the US, a difficult environment for the fostering of gender-equity claims. However, activists also found a way to make politicians and the general public personally connect with, and therefore care about, breast cancer as a major social problem.

Family erosion
The central means through which activists created a deeper sense of public concern about breast cancer was to frame the disease as a serious threat to American families, establishing a legitimate 'warrant' (Best 1987) for their demands of the federal government. While the construction of breast cancer as a female disease brought attention to the claim of gender equity, the construction of breast cancer as a threat to family stability highlighted the larger cultural importance of family in American politics and discourse in the 1990s. In the former construction of breast cancer as a problem of equity, women were portrayed as the sole victims of institutional neglect; in the latter, the pool of victims impacted by the disease expanded significantly to include the entire family. The expansion of the victim category had advantages for breast cancer activists. As Loseke (1999) has argued, the construction of a common

condition, one that casts the net wide enough to incorporate a larger number of victims, makes for a more successful claim. Publicly constructing breast cancer as a disease that threatened to erode families cast the net wide enough to incorporate breast cancer survivors and their families as victims of the disease.

In keeping with the claim that breast cancer threatened families, in public speech acts activists added family-based identities as wives and mothers to those of breast cancer survivor and advocate. Fran Visco's July 1992 introduction reflected the importance of constructing a family-based identity before Congress that privileged her identification as a wife and mother:

> Thank you. I am Fran Visco. I am a representative and the President of the National Breast Cancer Coalition. I am a mother, a wife and a breast cancer survivor (US Congress, Senate 21 July 1992: 487).

Beyond self-identification as wives or mothers, testimony often cast breast cancer victims in familial roles rather than simply as women. In one set of Nancy Brinker's testimony, she portrayed future victims of the disease primarily in familial roles:

> Another painful revelation for me to tell you is that in this decade, 1,600,000 women will be diagnosed with breast cancer. Five hundred thousand will die – mothers, grandmothers, sisters, daughters, friends – the list is endless (US Congress, Senate 20 June 1991: 13).

The typification of victims of breast cancer as female family members was also reflected in media accounts of the problem of funding for breast cancer research. On 30 May 1990, the *Washington Post* published a letter to the editor from an intern at the National Women's Health Network who characterised women who would die from the disease *as* family members:

> Breast cancer will strike an estimated 150,000 women in the United States this year. And it is estimated that more than 44,000 sisters, mothers, wives, daughters, and grand-daughters will die of breast cancer. Yet this year only 26 per cent of the National Cancer Institute's breast cancer grant requests have been approved because of lack of funds (*Washington Post*, 30 May 1990).

Along with the characterisation of breast cancer victims as female family members was an attribution of blame to the US government for the putative lack of National Cancer Institute (NCI) funding. From the perspective of the claimsmaker published in the *Post*, the following question was implicit: if the United States was losing 44,000 wives, mothers and daughters every year, why was the NCI not receiving increased research funding to lower this number? The more subtle accusation was that the annual loss of 44,000 female family members to breast cancer was directly linked to governmental neglect of the disease.

Typical claims of breast cancer as a threat to family stability also focused on the impact of the disease on husbands and children, the family members constructed as most affected by the incapacitation of a wife and mother. In detailing the story of her sister's treatment and ultimate death from breast cancer, Nancy Brinker testified as to the effects of the death of her sister on her surviving husband and child:

> She died three years later, after a painful bout with nine surgeries and three long, very, very painful sessions of chemotherapy. She left behind two young children, six and 10, a loving husband, and a family. Her absence has created, frankly, havoc in their lives (US Congress, Senate 20 June 1991: 11).

The construction of the devastating impact of 'motherloss' echoes a larger US cultural discourse that only women can provide children with a stable sense of self – that without mothers, children are deprived of an essential love only women can provide (Davidman 2001). Media accounts of the breast cancer epidemic also emphasised young, white women being taken away from 'loving families' (Lantz and Booth 1998), heightening panic about the disease. Activists drew on larger cultural concerns about 'family values' and the centrality of mothers to family stability to define the family as under attack by breast cancer. At times, activists directly relied on the discourse of family values to support their claim that breast cancer contributed to the breakdown of American families. Fran Visco's testimony made clear demands of Congress on the basis of family values rhetoric:

> Breast cancer destroys these women, and devastates their families. Politicians and the public can no longer merely pay lip service to the importance of family values. They must now act to halt the destruction of families devastated by this disease. Children lose their mothers, husbands lose their wives, brothers lose their sisters and parents lose their daughters to the epidemic of breast cancer (US Congress, Senate 29 July 1992: 488).

Despite individual political affiliations, the rhetoric of family values embedded in activist claims appealed to a bipartisan Congress and diverse public constituents. If increased funding for breast cancer would contribute to the stability of families, few could argue against this logic or demand.

The cultural power of breast cancer frames: frame viability versus validity

Though social constructionist accounts of social problems do not typically concern themselves with the validity of claims, the emphasis on frames as cultural resources in this case study lends itself to a consideration of the viability, versus the validity, of funding activist claims. This examination of frame validity is neither intended to debunk the claims of activists, nor detract from the importance of breast cancer research and women's health in the US. It does, however, illuminate the crucial sociological point that movement frames do not require 'validity' for successful claimsmaking, but rather must display a degree of cultural resonance, or cultural viability, with intended audiences to ensure strong public claims.

In the case of the epidemic frame, for example, breast cancer was defined in activist discourse as a widespread problem, a notion that was eventually challenged. As Lantz and Booth (1998) detail in their analysis of media framings of breast cancer in the US from 1980–1995, there has been disagreement about whether or not a true epidemic of breast cancer emerged in the 1980s. After reports of an increase in incidence were released and reiterated in media accounts, later studies suggested an association between higher breast cancer rates and the increased use of mammography rather than a real rise in incidence. Regardless of the validity of a breast cancer epidemic, the degree to which the notion of an epidemic saturated public opinion made for a culturally viable frame.

Likewise, the use of a gender-equity frame raises questions about both a national concern for women and cancer, and the history of funding for female cancers before the increases of the early 1990s. As noted previously, from the inception of the earliest cancer education campaigns in the US, women have been the primary targets for cancer education, screening and treatment (Leopold 1999, Lerner 2001, Rettig 1977, Ross 1987). The ACS was explicit in expressing a primary concern for female-related cancers: breast, uterine and ovarian cancer. Thus, historically, a public concern for women's cancers has always been at the forefront of voluntary associations. The GAO report outlining the NIH's neglect of women in clinical trials clearly raised the question of gender equity in government-funded health research, but in terms of funding cancer research, it was not necessarily the case that breast cancer had received unequal research funding at the NCI. In her study of breast cancer and chemical research in the US, Klawiter (2003) argues that breast cancer has consistently been at the forefront of cancer research planning agendas. In particular, Klawiter demonstrates that before the passage of the two major pieces of funding legislation of the early 1990s, breast cancer had actually received a greater portion of the NCI's total research budget than cancers that affected males more (*e.g.* prostate, lung) throughout the 1980s. As with the epidemic frame, the gender-equity frame – regardless of the validity of the claim that government was inequitably distributing funding resources – was effectively mobilised by breast cancer activists because of its strong cultural resonance. Rather than using male-related cancers as the counterpoint to allotments for breast cancer funding, activists instead referred to AIDS, coded in activist discourse as a gay male disease, as a central example of unequal research funding for women's health by government.

Breast cancer activists' appropriation of cancer frames

From a sociological perspective, the case of breast cancer funding activism is compelling because of its use of multiple, interconnected and culturally viable frames to demand increased federal funding for breast cancer research. And, while the rhetorical frames employed by breast cancer funding activists in the early 1990s are central to this analysis, their place within the larger context of cancer claimsmaking in the 20th century US highlights how social movements can appropriate and tailor prior movement frames for their specific cause. The framings of the breast cancer problem in the early 1990s represent the appropriation of previous definitions of the cancer problem for the purpose of narrowing categorical cancer research to breast cancer alone.

Past cancer advocacy efforts related to the establishment of, and increase in, federal funding for cancer research, for example, have used claims of high incidence rates and governmental responsibility for cancer. The two most significant pieces of public policy that resulted from such past efforts, including the concerns about a cancer epidemic, include FDR's establishment of the National Cancer Institute in 1937, and President Nixon's passage of the National Cancer Act of 1971 (Patterson 1987, Ross 1987). Like the rhetoric of breast cancer activists in the early 1990s, these prior cancer advocacy movements emphasised that the responsibility for funding biomedical research aimed at determining the cause, prevention and cure of cancer rested largely on the federal government, not private research foundations (Rettig 1977, Ross 1987). Thus, the idea that government should assume a large portion of the responsibility related to scientific knowledge about breast cancer reflected previous advocacy for cancer policy in general, but was utilised instead to highlight the importance of a single form of cancer.

Breast cancer funding activists also appropriated the frame of family erosion used in past cancer campaigns to reassign social responsibility for the disease from individual women to the federal government. The claim that cancer threatened families had long been a concern of cancer advocacy groups and public health campaigns, most notably the American Cancer Society (originally named the American Society for the Control of Cancer). The Women's Field Army established by the ACS in the 1930s explicitly targeted women as the audience for cancer education in private homes, in women's magazines and in women's clubs and organisations (Aronowitz 2001, Leopold 1999, Lerner 2001, Patterson 1987, Ross 1987). Defined in these efforts as the primary caretakers of family and family health, women's identities as wives and mothers have historically been utilised in cancer education campaigns.

Breast cancer funding activists built on these historical constructions of cancer as a threat to families, and the centrality of women to the stability of families, but flipped the definition of responsibility for such threats on its head. In previous iterations of the family erosion frame individual women were implicitly blamed for the threat of cancer to family stability. Neglecting to educate oneself about cancer, or to be proactive in the detection and treatment of the disease, was portrayed as antithetical to women's respons-ibilities as the gatekeepers for family health (Aronowitz 2001, Lerner 2001). According to past education campaigns, it was crucial for women to educate themselves about cancer in order to protect themselves and their families against the negative family impacts of the disease. Rather than focus on individual women's responsibility for cancer education and care, the 1990s iteration of the family erosion frame identified research funding as the primary problem of breast cancer and identified the federal government as centrally responsible for the continued problem of breast cancer. By employ-ing the family erosion frame with a new agenda and audience, activists, at a minimum, symbolically reassigned responsibility for breast cancer to the federal government and rejected the notion that individual women were responsible for the disease.

Having already been established by the media, the claim of a breast cancer epidemic allowed activists to redefine breast cancer from a problem of indi-vidual women to an urgent public health crisis. Activists utilised the rhetoric of an epidemic to define the repercussions of the disease as extending beyond individual women to a nation of women at risk, and to the larger economy, and demanded a governmental response. Activist use of of gender equity as the master frame aided the movement because of the strong cultural resonance, viability and past success of movement equity claims; it was also instrumental for contending that breast cancer was not receiving adequate federal funding. If the epidemic and gender-equity claims were not enough to stir compassion in the public audience of activist claims in the early 1990s, the family-erosion claim built the bridge that allowed for con-nection between abstract ideas of disparity, and the concrete experiences of breast cancer patients and their families. Government rhetoric in the early 1990s was heavily dominated by the discourse of family values, and the family-erosion claim drew upon this cultural and political opportunity to increase the resonance of the movement's demands. Any one of these frames alone may not have been as viable as the combination of the three in the public domain. While sometimes contradictory, particularly in terms of the messages they sent about gender, the three frames worked symbiotically to construct an urgent situation that affected a socially marginalised group valued for the stability they provided to families.

Conclusion: cultural resources in social movements: the importance of framing

By analysing the rhetorical discourse of breast cancer funding activism in the early 1990s, this analysis builds on recent sociological interest in the cultural aspects of HSMs specifically, and social movements generally. In particular, I argue that an important component of the breast cancer movement's efforts to attain increased funding in the early 1990s was its use of culturally resonant and *viable* frames in discursive activities to connect with, and persuade, public audiences. This study makes no claims as to whether or not the frames themselves caused increases in funding. Future research might be able to assess this causal relationship if it takes the approach of recent studies that analyse the effects of claims on health policymaking (Lantz, Weisman and Itani 2003). And though much social movement research focuses on the mobilisation of structural resources, this chapter demonstrates the importance of taking into account the culturally viable resources mobilised by HSMs, building on an ongoing line of research on culture and social movements (Johnston and Klandermans 1995, Poletta 1997, Swidler 1986, 1995).

The findings of this study raise questions about how other health social movements might fare in terms of the cultural resources they bring to, or draw upon, in their efforts. Breast cancer, for example, is often considered an ideal cause in part because few could oppose the goal of finding a cure for the disease. In addition, there has been a great deal of public attention to the disease in the past 30 years. In the context of this study, breast cancer funding activism was compelling because of its use of multiple, culturally resonant and viable frames. Other diseases, however, may have more limited cultural resources, including viable frames, that could result in less public attention and resources than breast cancer.

The ability of other health movements to attain public resources may depend on how easily they can appropriate the resonant frames of other successful health social movements. The claim of gender equity, for example, appears to have had less resonance in other health movements. Prostate cancer in the US, for example, has succeeded in increasing its total research monies in the past decade, but nowhere near the amount the funding levels of breast cancer. In part, this lack of comparable funding may be due to a less viable gender-equity claim in the public sphere. Prostate cancer advocates have claimed that 'true' gender equities can be seen in prostate cancer funding – which receives more total funding than breast cancer – but represents a disease that affects men at a rate similar to that of breast cancer in women. To date, these arguments have not resulted in equal funding levels. It may be that equity claims resonated more strongly with the public when used on behalf of women, a more recognisable minority group than men.

In addition, the equity and epidemic frames may have a shorter shelf life than expected in the realm of biomedical research activism. If equity claims and the use of incidence statistics become standard in health social movement efforts to demand public funding, the frames themselves could lose cultural viability potency. With increased resources for any one disease, inequity will automatically be created for others; there could be no end to health movement claims that specific diseases are not addressed equitably by government. The question becomes which health social movements will be successfully able to define their situations as inequitable, how long such frames can retain cultural viability, and which movements will have to develop new frames to increase governmental resources.

Second, other health social movements may be limited by the social value of the group of victims it portrays. The epidemic frame appropriated by funding activists portrayed breast cancer not just as affecting a large number of women, but presenting a particular threat to young, white, middle class women (Lantz and Booth 1998). Thus, other health social movements might bring fewer cultural resources to their activities in terms of the social value of the victims portrayed in accounts of their cause, impacting upon their ability to convince audiences that their disease is a serious public problem.

Similarly, other health movements may have fewer cultural resources to draw upon if their condition has a strong social stigma that prevents it from being defined as a problem of governmental policy. Obesity, for example, could be defined as the fault of government due to food policies and the reduction in physical education programmes in public schools (Critser 2003), but such efforts would probably be less successful than those of breast cancer activists. Despite recent media attention to the social and political factors related to obesity in the US, public discourse largely places the onus for obesity on individuals and their inability to control eating behaviours.

Other health social movements may also be enhanced or limited by activism that preceded their efforts. In the case of breast cancer, activists were able to draw upon and appropriate frames from past cancer advocacy that had a strong history of success in US health policymaking. Without question, the breast cancer movement also benefited from the past efforts of the women's health movement and the AIDS movement, resulting in 'social movement spillover' (Epstein 1996, Meyer and Whittier 1994). Past activist efforts may not be necessary for health social movements to construct viable claims, but in some cases may make it easier for movements to pursue specific goals from a broader base of public interest in a disease.

Importantly, the focus on the US raises questions about how breast cancer funding might vary across national contexts. Both Canada and the UK have developed 'sister' breast cancer activist coalitions (Breast Cancer Action and the UK National Breast Cancer Coalition) and have succeeded in increasing the amount of governmental funds earmarked for breast cancer research. On the surface, however, some variations might reveal differences in the structural or cultural contexts of funding activism. Both British and Canadian research initiatives and funds are constituted by combined corporate/private, philanthropic and governmental sources which suggests more private/public partnerships for research funding that could in turn shape how advocates identify 'responsible' parties. In addition, the amount of money for such funding is far lower than that provided by the US government. While this might be due to smaller populations, the US could be unique in its large funding of diseases.

This case study also speaks to the important role of frames and framing processes in the study of social movements generally. Specifically, this study builds on recent scholarship in the cultural study of social movements that argues for the inclusion of frames as a cultural resource used by social movement actors to pursue their goals (Williams 1995). From this perspective, frames, as 'cultural tool kits' (Swidler 1986, Taylor and Whittier 1995, Williams and Benford 2000), are as central to the processes of social movements as political opportunities, networks and institutional relationships. Examining the cultural resonance of frames naturally complements structural analyses of social movements.

The issue of frame viability versus validity has also been central to the analysis of frames in this study. From a subjectivist viewpoint, frames need not be accurate or verifiable to become successful in the public sphere. Instead, the cultural viability of frames appears to carry more weight in some social movements than others. Movements that employ frames with high cultural viability may succeed more than movements representing people with high morbidity and mortality.

This chapter also demonstrates how frames can be used by social movements not only for increased material resources, but also for the purpose of 'frame transformation' (Snow *et al.* 1986), or the redefinition of social conditions. In the case of breast cancer, funding activists used the epidemic, gender equity and family-erosion frames to redefine breast cancer from a private problem of individual women to a public problem of governmental neglect. On a symbolic level, social movement framing processes actively create meaning about social conditions, often in opposition to dominant conceptions. It is not just movement activities themselves, (*e.g.* picketing, lobbying, testifying, marching), but also the definitions of conditions expressed through such actions that transform public understandings of social conditions. And while individual women are still implicitly blamed for breast cancer in media accounts (Brown *et al.* 2001), for a time activist discourse defined breast cancer as a problem of governmental neglect, even if only symbolically.

Last, this case study demonstrates that some social movements can employ multiple, and sometimes contradictory, frames in their discursive activities. Indeed, breast cancer funding activists employed three frames, two of which sent contradictory messages about gender. On the one hand, activists used the gender-equity frame to define themselves as part of an angry disenfranchised group that would not stay silent in the face of governmental neglect. On the other hand, activists also employed the family-erosion frame that defined women primarily in familial roles of wives and mothers, and asked the state to protect them as the natural centres of stability for families. While the gender-equity claim rang of a feminist approach to social change, the family-erosion claim reinforced traditional notions of white, middle class, heterosexual motherhood. Taylor and Whittier (1995) found that self-help movements often embodied contradictory gender frames, challenging dominant ideologies of gender, while reinforcing others. Though at times contradictory, activists successfully used three frames simultaneously to define breast cancer as a major social problem. This suggests that other social movements may also use more than one frame in their discursive activities to varying effects.

HSM activism related to access to health care and health services has not necessarily been pushed aside by recent HSMs, but at times is approached through the newer route of federally-funded, disease-specific research activism. Concerns for quality healthcare remain central to funding activism, but are increasingly addressed through scientific means. Indeed, the stated purpose of improved disease-specific research is that the expansion of scientific knowledge will lead to better treatments, better methods of prevention and perhaps the elimination of the necessity for care in the first place if disease can be 'eradicated' through science. These represent high hopes, and no doubt reflect the high cultural value placed on scientific knowledge in the US, but the quest for better healthcare and health services will continue to be pursued by HSMs – one claim and one research dollar at a time.

Acknowledgments

I would like to thank the anonymous reviewers; the special issue editors, Phil Brown and Stephen Zavestoski; and the monograph editor at *Sociology of Health & Illness* for their invaluable comments. I also want to thank Peter Conrad, Jennifer Ginsburg Richard, Jean Elson, Heather T. Jacobson, Sandi Kawecka Nenga, Valerie Leiter, Brent Stephens and Stefan Timmermans for providing the feedback necessary for the development of this chapter.

Notes

1   Other scholars have written about the scientific dimensions of breast cancer activism in the 1990s (Epstein 1996, Myhre 2001), but this analysis aims to specify the character of 'funding activism' as a subset of what Epstein terms 'treatment activism' or 'scientific activism'.

2   Though this analysis uses a social constructionist approach to examine discursive rhetoric as a cultural resource for HSM demands, it by no means discounts the importance of broader social and political contexts for such success. This analysis takes into account the rhetoric of this movement period, complementing Weisman's (2000) structural analysis of breast cancer policymaking throughout the 1990s.

3   The term 'elite core' is used to reflect the character of the NBCC – the primary, publicly recognised claimsmaker. While there is no single breast cancer movement (Boehmer 2000, Klawiter 1999b, Myhre 2001, Taylor and Van Willigen 1996), this chapter focuses on the group of activists who received the most governmental and media attention at the time – mostly white, middle to upper class heterosexual women (Myhre 2001).

4   Epstein (1996, 1997) details the development of varied 'genocide' claims as the AIDS movement developed. Though breast cancer activists did not use the direct language of genocide, implicit in this testimony is the notion that a social group is in danger of extinction.

5   Ironically, despite the efforts and successes of AIDS activists to culturally redefine AIDS as a disease that puts all citizens at risk (Epstein 1996), breast cancer

activists relied on male-centred definitions of the disease to bolster their claims of gender *in*equity in the allocation of federal monies.

6   The issue of gendered expressions of emotion in public is relevant to the public testimonies of breast cancer activists. Montini's study of informed consent legislation (1996) found that advocates relied on emotions of fear and grief, stereotypical definitions of appropriate female expression, in order to ensure that their arguments were heard in the legislative arena. Mainstream breast cancer activism in the early 1990s has been characterised as non-contentious in their lobbying efforts compared to the AIDS movement (Epstein 1996, Myhre 2001), but the data collected for this chapter suggest that there was a notable shift from the expression of stereotypically female emotions to stereotypically non-female emotion – anger – in public testimony. Perhaps the breast cancer movement of the early 1990s lies conceptually between contentious and consensus movements. Most interestingly, these funding activists engaged in the public expression of anger while simultaneously appealing to the state on the basis of family values, appealing to the conservative notion that mothers are central to family stability.

References

Altman, R. (1996) *Waking up/Fighting back: the Politics of Breast Cancer*. Boston, MA: Little, Brown and Company.

Anglin, M.K. (1997) Working from the inside out: implications of breast cancer activism for biomedical policies and practices, *Social Science and Medicine*, 44, 9, 1403–15.

Aronowitz, R. (2001) 'Do not delay': breast cancer and time, 1900–1970, *The Milbank Quarterly*, 79, 3, 355–86.

Benford, R.D. and Hunt, S.A. (1995) Dramaturgy and social movements: the social construction and communication of power. In Lyman, S.M. (ed.) *Social Movements: Critiques, Concepts, Case-Studies*. New York: New York University Press.

Benford, R.D. and Snow, D.A. (2000) Framing processes and social movements: an overview and assessment, *Annual Review of Sociology*, 26, 611–39.

Best, J. (1987) Rhetoric in claims-making: constructing the missing children problem, *Social Problems*, 34, 2, 101–21.

Best, J. (1995) Constructionism in context. In Best, J. (ed.) *Images of Issues: Typifying Contemporary Social Problems*. New York: Aldine de Gruyter.

Boehmer, U. (2000) *The Personal and the Political: Women's Activism in Response to the Breast Cancer and AIDS Epidemics*. New York: State University of New York Press.

Boonstra, H. (1990) Trivialising women's health, *Washington Post*, 30th May.

Brown, P., Zavestoski, S.M., McCormick, S., Mandelbaum, J. and Luebke, T. (2001) Print media coverage of environmental causes of breast cancer, *Sociology of Health and Illness*, 23, 6, 747–75.

Brown, P., Zavestoski, S., McCormick, S. and Mayer, B. (2002) Health Social Movements: Uncharted Territory in Social Movement Research, paper presented as part of the Collective Behavior and Social Movement Section of the American Sociological Association, Chicago, IL., August 2002.

Critser, G. (2003) *Fat Land: how Americans Became the Fattest People in the World*. Boston: Houghton Mifflin Company.

Davidman, L. (2001) *Motherloss*. Berkeley, CA: University of California Press.

Epstein, S. (1996) *Impure Science: AIDS, Activism, and the Politics of Knowledge*. Berkeley: University of California Press.

Epstein, S. (1997) AIDS activism and the retreat from the 'genocide' frame, *Social Identities*, 3, 3, 415–38.

Ferraro, S. (1993) The anguished politics of breast cancer. *New York Times Magazine*, 15 August, 6, 21.

Fine, G.A. (1995) Public narration and group culture: discerning discourse in social movements. In Johnston, H. and Klandermans, B. (eds) *Social Movements and Culture*. Minneapolis: University of Minnesota Press.

Freligh, R. (1993) Breast cancer her crusade. *Plain Dealer*, 7 September 1993, Pg. 1F.

Goffman, E. (1974) *Frame Analysis: An Essay on the Organization of Experience*. Boston: Northeastern University Press.

Giugni, M.G. (1998) Was it worth the effort? The outcomes and consequences of social movements, *Annual Review of Sociology*, 98, 371–93.

Hilgartner, S.H. and Bosk, C.L. (1988) The rise and fall of social problems: a public arenas model, *American Journal of Sociology*, 94, 1, 53–78.

Johnston, H. (1995) A methodology for frame analysis: from discourse to cognitive schemata. In Johnston, H. and Klandermans, B. (eds) *Social Movements and Culture*. Minneapolis: University of Minnesota Press.

Johnston, H. and Klandermans, B. (eds) (1995) *Social Movements and Culture*. Minneapolis: University of Minnesota Press.

Johnston, H., Laraña, E. and Gusfield, J.R. (1994) Identities, grievances, and new social movements. In Johnston, L. and Gusfield (eds) *New Social Movements: from Ideology to Identity*. Philadelphia: Temple University Press.

Johnston, H. and Klandermans, B. (1995) The cultural analysis of social movements. In Johnston, H. and Klandermans, B. (eds) *Social Movements and Culture*. Minneapolis: University of Minnesota Press.

Klawiter, M. (1999a) *Reshaping the Contours of Breast Cancer: from Private Stigma to Public Actions*. Ph.D. dissertation, Department of Sociology, University of California, Berkeley.

Klawiter, M. (1999b) Racing for the cure, walking women, and toxic touring: mapping cultures of action within the Bay Area terrain of breast cancer, *Social Problems*, 46, 1, 104–26.

Klawiter, M. (2003) Chemicals, cancer, and prevention: the synergy of synthetic social movements. In Casper, M. (ed.) *Synthetic Planet: Chemical Politics and the Hazards of Modern Life*. New York: Routledge.

Lantz, P.M. and Booth, K.M. (1998) The social construction of the breast cancer epidemic, *Social Science & Medicine*, 46, 7, 907–18.

Lantz, P.M., Weisman, C.S. and Itani, Z. (2003) A disease-specific Medicaid expansion for women: The Breast and Cervical Cancer Prevention and Treatment Act of 2000, *Women's Health Issues*, 13, 79–92.

Leopold, E. (1999) *A Darker Ribbon: Breast Cancer, Women, and their Doctors in the Twentieth Century*. Boston, MA: Beacon Press Books.

Lerner, B.H. (2001) *The Breast Cancer Wars: Hope, Fear, and the Pursuit of a Cure in Twentieth-Century America*. New York: Oxford University Press.

Loseke, D. (1999) *Thinking About Social Problems: an Introduction to Constructionist Perspectives*. New York: Aldine de Gruyter.

Love, S.M. and Lindsey, K. (1997) The politics of breast cancer. In Richardson, L., Taylo, V. and Whittier, N. (eds) *Feminist Frontiers IV*. New York: McGraw Hill.

Love, S.M. (1993) Breast cancer what the department of defense should do with its $210 million, *Journal of the American Medical Association*, 269, 18, 2417.

McAdam, D. (1994) Culture and social movements. In Johnston, L. and Gusfield, J.K. (eds) *New Social Movements: from Ideology to Identity*. Philadelphia: Temple University Press.

Meyer, D.S. and Whittier, N. (1994) Social movement spillover, *Social Problems*, 41, 277–98.

Mills, C. Wright (1959) *The Sociological Imagination*. New York: Oxford University Press.

Mirola, W.A. (2003) Asking for bread, receiving a stone: the rise and fall of religious ideologies in Chicago's eight-hour movement, *Social Problems*, 50, 2, 273–93.

Montini, T. (1996) Gender and emotion in the advocacy for breast cancer informed consent legislation, *Gender and Society*, 10, 1, 9–23.

Myhre, J. (2001) Medical mavens: gender, science, and the consensus politics of breast cancer. Ph.D dissertation, University of California, Davis.

Patterson, J.T. (1987) *The Dread Disease: Cancer and Modern American Culture*. Cambridge, MA: Harvard University Press.

Polletta, F. (1997) Culture and its discontents: recent theorizing on the cultural dimensions of protest, *Sociological Inquiry*, 67, 4, 431–50.

Reese, E. and Newcombe, G. (2003) Income rights, mothers' rights, or workers' rights? Collective action frames, organizational ideologies, and the American Welfare Rights Movement, *Social Problems*, 50, 2, 294–318.

Rettig, R.A. (1977) *Cancer Crusade: the Story of the National Cancer Act of 1971*. Princeton, NJ: Princeton University Press.

Ross, W.S. (1987) *Crusade: the Official History of the American Cancer Society*. New York: Arbor House.

Scott, J. and Love, S. (1993) Setting the agenda for the politics of breast cancer. *Los Angeles Times*, 5 December 1993, Part M., 3, Opinion Desk.

Simpson, C. (2000) Controversies in breast cancer prevention: the discourse of risk. In Potts, L.K. (ed.) *Ideologies of Breast Cancer: Feminist Perspectives*. New York: St. Martin's Press, Inc.

Snow, D.A., Rochford Jr., E.B., Worden, S.K. and Benford, R.D. (1986) Frame alignment processes, micromobilization, and movement participation, *American Sociological Review*, 51, 464–81.

Snow, D.A. and Benford, R.D. (1992) Master Frames and Cycles of Protest. In Morris, A.D. and Mueller, C.M. (eds) *Frontiers in Social Movement Theory*. New Haven, CT: Yale University Press.

Spector, M. and Kitsuse, J.I. (1977) *Constructing Social Problems*. Menlo Park, CA: Cummings Publishing Company.

Swidler, A. (1986) Culture in action: symbols and strategies, *American Sociological Review*, 51, 273–86.

Swidler, A. (1995) Cultural power and social movements. In Johnston, H. and Klandermans, B. (eds) *Social Movements and Culture*. Minneapolis: University of Minnesota Press.

Tarrow, S. (1992) Mentalities, political cultures, and collective action frames: constructing meaning through action. In Morris, A.D. and Mueller, C.M. (ed.) *Frontiers in Social Movement Theory*. New Haven, CT: Yale University Press.

Taylor, V. and Whittier, N. (1995) Analytical approaches to social movement culture: the culture of the women's movement. In Johnston, H. and Klandermans, B. (eds) *Social Movements and Culture*. Minneapolis: University of Minnesota Press.

Taylor, V. and Van Willigen, M. (1996) Women's self-help and the reconstruction of gender: the postpartum support and breast cancer movements, *Mobilization*, 1, 2, 123–42.

Weisman, C.S. (2000) Breast cancer policymaking. In Kasper, A.S. and Ferguson, S.J. (eds) *Breast Cancer: Society Shapes an Epidemic*. New York: St. Martin's Press.

Williams, R.H. (1995) Constructing the public good: social movements and cultural resources, *Social Problems*, 42, 1, 124–44.

Williams, R.H. and Benford, R.D. (2000) Two faces of collective action frames: a theoretical consideration, *Current Perspectives in Social Theory* 20, 127–51.

Williams, G.I. and Williams, R.H. (1995) 'All We Want is Equality': rhetorical framing in the Father's Rights Movement. In Best, J. (ed.) *Images of Issues: Typifying Contemporary Social Problems*. New York: Walter de Gruyter, Inc.

Wuthnow, R. (1989) *Communities of Discourse: Ideology and Social Structure in the Reformation, the Enlightenment, and European Socialism*. Cambridge, MA: Harvard University Press.

Government Documents

US Congress. Senate. Committee on Aging. *Breast Cancer: Race for the Cure: Hearing Before the Subcommittee on Health and Long-Term Care of the Select Committee on Aging*. 101st Cong., 2nd sess., 16 May 1990.

US Congress. Senate. Committee on Labor and Human Resources. *Twentieth Anniversary of the National Cancer Act: Hearing Before the Committee on Labor and Human Resources*. 102nd Cong., 1st sess., 25 April 1991.

US Congress. Senate. Committee on Labor and Human Resources. *Why Are We Losing the War on Breast Cancer? Hearing Before the Subcommittee on Aging of the Committee on Labor and Human Resources*. 102nd Cong., 1st sess., 20 June 1991.

US Congress. Senate. Committee on Government Operations. *Breast Cancer Research and Treatment: Progress and Failures in the 20-Year War on Breast Cancer: Hearing before the Human Resources and Intergovernmental Relations*. 102nd Cong., 1st sess., 11 December 1991.

US Congress. Senate. Committee on Labor and Human Resources. *Combating the Rising Incidence of Breast Cancer: Prevention, Early Detection, and Treatment: Hearing of the Committee on Labor and Human Resources*. 102nd Cong., 2nd sess., 4 May 1992.

US Congress. Senate. Committee on Appropriations. *Departments of Labor, Health and Human Services, and Education, and Related Agencies Appropriations for Fiscal Year 1993: Hearings before a Subcommittee of the Committee on Appropriations*. 102nd Cong., 2nd sess., 28–30th July 1992.

US Congress. Senate. Select Committee on Aging. *Breast Cancer: Winning the Battles, Losing the War: Joint Hearing Before the Select Committee on Aging and the Subcommittee on Health and Long-Term Care*. 102nd Cong., 2nd sess., 1 October 1992.

Chapter 9

Breast cancer in two regimes: the impact of social movements on illness experience
Maren Klawiter

Introduction

This chapter uses the narrative of one woman, Clara Larson, to explore changes over time in the experiences of illness available to women diagnosed with breast cancer. To claim that different illness experiences become available at different times is simply to acknowledge that experiences of disease are shaped not only by the individual circumstances of disease sufferers and the particular character of their pathologies, but by culturally, spatially and historically specific regimes of practices. The regime of breast cancer has undergone a series of dramatic changes over the course of the last three decades and these changes are, in large part, the result of social movements. This chapter examines the impact of social movements on the regime of breast cancer and experiences of illness, paying particular attention to the ways in which gender and sexuality are constituted within disease regimes and challenged by social movements.

Clara Larson (not her real name) was 56 years old when I interviewed her in the San Francisco Bay Area in 1998. A white, middle class lesbian, divorced, a feminist, and the mother of four adult children, Clara Larson was first diagnosed with breast cancer in 1979, at the age of 37, and then again in 1997. Her narrative thus provides a window onto changes over time in the regime of breast cancer. There is nothing about Clara Larson that is ordinary or average. Likewise, the field of social movements in the San Francisco Bay Area is in no way representative of any other region or arena of activism. I view these anomalies as analytic assets, however, not as disadvantages. Clara's lesbian identity and feminist sensibilities constitute an 'outsider within' perspective (Collins 1999) that helps illuminate the ways in which gender and sexuality were embedded, embodied, imposed and exercised within the Bay Area regime of breast cancer. In like fashion, the depth and dynamism of the Bay Area field of activism helps reveal the remarkable extent to which disease regimes and illness experiences can be reshaped by social movements.

Between the early 1970s, when Clara received her first screening mammogram, and the late 1990s, when Clara was diagnosed with metastatic disease, an important set of changes took place in the regime of breast cancer. During the 1970s and 1980s, controversies over specific medical practices – mammographic screening, informed consent, the 'one-step' procedure and the radical mastectomy – resulted in specific changes in the regime of practices (see

Bailar 1976, Rennie 1977, Kushner 1977a, 1977b, 1986, Ross 1987, Montini and Ruzek 1989, Montini and Slobin 1991, Montini 1996, 1997, Leopold 1999, Lerner 2000, 2001, Weisman 2000, Centers for Disease Control and Prevention 2000). Some of these changes were tied to Consensus Development Conferences held by the National Institutes of Health (NIH). Others were codified in state and federal legislation. For the most part, however, the breast cancer activism of the 1970s and 1980s consisted of small, narrowly targeted and fleeting mobilisations fed by the ideologies, networks, and sometimes the organisations of pre-existing social movements – feminism, the women's health movement, the patients' rights movement and the consumer movement (see for example Montini 1996, 1997). The changes inspired by these targeted mobilisations were important, but they did not result in the formation of a breast cancer movement with its own organisations, activists, analysis, identity and agenda (Klawiter 1999b: 57–69, Leopold 1999: 188–214).

What changed during the 1990s was the scale and scope of breast cancer activism. These changes included the rapid growth in the number, size and funding of women's cancer and breast cancer organisations; the development of new discourses, cognitive frameworks and other forms of cultural production; the proliferation of new projects, campaigns and coalitions; and the cross-fertilisation of the breast cancer and environmental movements. A great deal has already been written about the history of the National Breast Cancer Coalition (NBCC) and its tremendous success in the federal legislative and policy-making arenas – lobbying to increase federal spending on breast cancer research, promoting the expansion of breast cancer screening programmes for low-income women, and gaining a 'seat at the table' where research funding decisions were being made (see especially Ferraro 1993, Dickersin and Schnaper 1996, Weisman 2000). The popular media attention generated by the NBCC no doubt contributed a great deal to the US public's growing awareness and support of the breast cancer movement. But the NBCC was not an important player in the San Francisco Bay Area field of social movements, where I conducted my research between 1994 and 1998. What I discovered instead was a dynamic 'field of contention' (Crossly 1998, 2003) fed by a diverse assortment of organisations that coalesced into three different 'cultures of action' (Klawiter 1999a, 1999b).

Each of these cultures of action challenged and changed the Bay Area regime of breast cancer. The success of these challenges was evident in the thoroughly transformed public discourses, emotional vocabularies, popular images and collective identities through which breast cancer – at least for urban, middle class white women in the San Francisco Bay Area – was navigated, negotiated, interpreted and experienced. This occurred through the efforts of mainstream organisations such as the Susan G. Komen Breast Cancer Foundation and its signature event, Race for the Cure®, which attracted thousands of participants to Golden Gate Park every year (beginning in 1991) to celebrate the beauty, strength and enduring femininity of 'breast cancer survivors', to raise money for medical research and to fund mobile mammography vans to provide mammograms to low-income women. The mainstream movement was so successful in transforming the public discourse of breast cancer that leading names in corporate America, especially the beauty, fitness and fashion industries, adopted breast cancer as their *cause celebre*[1]. These developments had a significant impact on the regime of breast cancer. Breast cancer awareness ribbons (pink), pins, T-shirts, cosmetics, clothing, shoes, athletic gear, fashion shows, walk-a-thons, swim-a-thons, races, hikes, climbs and other public events and campaigns challenged the architecture of the closet that had confined earlier generations. The mainstream breast cancer awareness movement replaced the stigmatisation, isolation and invisibility of women with breast cancer with a new public culture overflowing with symbolic gestures of support, solidarity, respect and recognition. The public identity of women with breast cancer was transformed from tragic victim to heroic survivor. The public image of the new breast cancer survivor, unlike the victim of yesteryear, was a woman whose femininity, sexuality and desirability were intact; a woman who had struggled bravely and victoriously against the disease (which, ideally, was diagnosed early, due to her disciplined practice of 'breast health' and rigorous observation of screening guidelines), and whose survival was therefore assured. Gender and sexuality were intimately bound up in these social and cultural transformations.

In addition to the more mainstream, corporatised wing of the breast cancer movement, lesbian, feminist and environmental activists politicised the issue of breast cancer in the San Francisco Bay Area. A number of organisations were involved in this effort. The oldest of the bunch, the Women's Cancer Resource Center, was founded in 1986 by Jackie Winnow, a feminist, lesbian and AIDS activist. In 1990, Breast Cancer Action, a pioneering feminist treatment activist organisation, was founded by a group of women who met in a support group for women with metastatic breast cancer. In 1991, the Breast Cancer Fund was founded by Andrea Martin, a businesswoman and a feminist twice diagnosed with breast cancer. That same year, inspired by AIDS activism, three lesbians founded the Women and Cancer Project to raise money for local organisations. The Charlotte Maxwell Complementary Clinic, founded in 1991, provided free alternative and complementary cancer therapies to low-income women. In 1994, feminist cancer organisations teamed up with environmental justice organisations and created the Toxic Links Coalition, a synthesis of the two which quickly expanded to include a wide-range of environmental and cancer organisations. Inspired by the activism of the Toxic Links Coalition, Marin Breast Cancer Watch, an environmental breast cancer organisation, was founded in 1995.

Feminist and environmental breast cancer activism in the San Francisco Bay Area operated along multiple dimensions – providing free services, support and complementary therapies to women with cancer, staging public events, political protests, educational forums and art exhibits, lobbying the state legislature for breast cancer research funding and greater access to breast cancer screening and treatment for low-income women. Feminist breast cancer activism also challenged the optimistic narratives, images and emotional displays of the mainstream movement. In this culture of action, women with histories of breast cancer were more likely to speak of 'living with cancer' than being a 'survivor'. Many women with mastectomies did not wear breast prostheses and, rejecting the idea of putting a pretty bow on an ugly reality, they rarely wore pink ribbons – though many wore the 'Cancer Sucks' buttons designed by Breast Cancer Action. They were sceptical of the effectiveness of mammographic screening, angry at the government and critical of the medical research establishment.

Feminist cancer organisations in the San Francisco Bay Area had, since their inception, promoted an environmental analysis of breast cancer. This focus intensified during the second half of the 1990s, as the feminist cancer and environmental movements began working together on a number of different projects (see Klawiter 2003). Some organisations, like The Breast Cancer Fund, organized a Bay Area environmental study group and sponsored research on breast cancer and the environment. Others, like the Toxic Links Coalition, Breast Cancer Action and the Women's Cancer Resource Center, were more oriented toward direct action and public protests. Marin Breast Cancer Watch embarked upon its own research projects, for which it eventually secured funding from the state (of California). Overall, this organisational field shared a common goal of linking the growing incidence of breast cancer (and cancer generally speaking) to environmental pollution and corporate profits.

Elsewhere, I have emphasised the differences between mainstream, feminist and environmental activism in the Bay Area, but here I want simply to recognise their collective impact on the regime of breast cancer and the illness experiences available to women residing within and passing through it. Certainly, these changes were not experienced in the same way or to the same degree by every woman. Subject positions and social locations – age, race, class, culture, ethnicity, sexual identity, religion and political convictions – also shaped women's relationship to the regime of breast cancer. But every woman diagnosed with breast cancer in the Bay Area during the late 1990s encountered a different set of conditions – a different regime of practices – than that encountered by the generations that preceded them.

The remainder of this chapter is organised as follows: in the next section, I locate this study within the scholarship on illness experience, develop the concept of disease regime and explore the relationship between disease regimes, social movements and illness experience. A section on research data and methods follows. I then proceed to the heart of the matter, the illness experience of Clara Larson. Divided into two parts – 1979 and 1997 – Larson's narrative focuses our attention on key changes over time in the regime of breast cancer and the impact of social movements on her illness experience. I conclude with some reflections on the contributions of this study to the current state of theorising about illness experience.

Disease regimes, illness experience and social movements

In a recent review of the literature on illness experience, Janine Pierret (2003) identifies 'the social structure' as 'the problem to be analyzed' (2003: 17). Pierret calls for research that moves beyond the simple examination of structural factors in order to show how these structural factors actually shape the illness experience (2003: 15). Pierret also identifies the role of patient organisations as one of the key areas in which 'work remains to be done' (2003: 16) and she calls for new paradigms that work out the interrelationships between social structures, cultural factors and subjective experience. This chapter responds to Pierret's call for new research and frameworks that address the relationship between social structures and illness experience. It also responds to Pierret's call for more research on the role of patient organisations. In place of patient organisations, however, I broaden the focus to social movements. In place of social structures I analyse disease regimes.

The concept of disease regime is derived from Foucault's (1987) 'regime of practices'. Foucault uses this term to refer to an apparatus of practices organised around a shared problematic. In *Discipline and Punish* (1979) for example, Foucault analysed regimes of punishment. In *History of Sexuality* (1978), he analysed modern sexuality. In both instances – and in his historical investigations of madness (1965), public health (1980) and medicine (1973) – the 'target of analysis', as Foucault puts it, 'wasn't "institutions," "theories," or "ideology," but *practices*' (1987: 102). Within Foucault's framework of analysis, practices 'are not just governed by institutions, prescribed by ideologies, guided by pragmatic circumstances – whatever role these elements may actually play – but possess up to a point their own specific regularities, logic, strategy, self-evidence, and "reason"' (1987: 103). Ultimately, as Foucault argues, the task of the investigator (or genealogist) is the analysis of these regimes. Although Foucault repeatedly claims that 'where there is power, there is resistance', he focuses his own analysis on power, not resistance.

Scholars such as Robert Castel (1991), David Armstrong (1993, 1995), Deborah Lupton (1995), Alan Petersen (1997, with Lupton 1996) and Robin Bunton (with Burrows 1995, with Petersen 1997) have drawn on Foucault with great success in their research on regimes of public health and medicine. This chapter is indebted to the work of these scholars. But as is the case in Foucault's own work, scholarship in this tradition tends to portray regimes of public health and medicine in rather totalising terms. In part, this is because the lived experience of health and illness – 'history from below' in Roy Porter's (1985) terms – is largely absent from the analysis. In part, it is because social movements and other forms of collectively organised resistance are not foregrounded. The concept of disease regime, as I deploy it here, draws on the insights of this Foucauldan tradition but departs from its totalising view of power.

Some disease regimes are totalising, others less so. Some regimes are anchored in multiple institutions. Others are less expansive. Although they are relatively structured and stable, disease regimes are subject to a wide variety of cross-cutting pressures. Some of these pressures originate within the powerful industries and institutions in which they are anchored – the healthcare, insurances and pharmaceutical industries, for example, as well as the institutions of science, medicine, the state, popular culture and the media. Others originate in the non-establishment approaches of medically marginalised traditions – folk medicine, alternative treatment modalities, unorthodox science and non-Western epistemologies of health, disease and the body[2]. Still others originate in the counternarratives and practices of social movements. All of these are important, but this chapter focuses on those forces of change that originate in social movements.

In my formulation, disease regimes are comprised of the institutionalised practices, authoritative discourses, social relations, collective identities, emotional vocabularies, visual images, public policies and regulatory actions through which diseases are socially constituted and experienced. Because social movements are capable of affecting each and every one of these dimensions, they can have profoundly transformative effects on disease regimes. Not all social movements are equally powerful, of course, nor do all social movements work along each and every one of these dimensions. Some social movements target the formal political arena, impacting public policy, regulatory practices and judicial decisions. Others achieve their greatest impact in the cultural arena, changing the popular images, ideas, emotions and identities associated with a particular disease, creating new representations and alternative ways of seeing and experiencing the disease and constructing new collective identities. Other social movements ('self-help' movements, for example) achieve their greatest impact by altering the social relations of disease – creating new social spaces, networks, scripts and subjectivities – changing the sick role and social interactions with friends, family, physicians and even strangers. Even social movements that do not change specific practices within a disease regime can have an impact on an individual's illness experience by transforming her perceptions of, and relationship to, practices of the regime.

Finally, we know that all social institutions are shaped by, and shape, gender and sexuality (Connel 1987, Lorber 1994). We know that illness experiences are mediated by gender (Ruzek 1978, Doyal 1995, Lorber 1997). And we know that gender is a pervasive feature of social movements (see especially Taylor 1999, also Brown and Ferguson 1995, Ferree and Martin 1995, Gamson 1997, Ferree and Roth 1998, Fonow 1998, Naples 1998, Ray 1998, 1999, Klawiter 1999a). This chapter builds on this foundation by exploring the ways in which gender and sexuality are constituted within different regimes of breast cancer, shape illness experiences, and are challenged by social movements.

Data and methods

Clara Larson's illness narrative is foregrounded in this chapter, but my method is not that of narrative analysis (see Lawton 2003, Pierret 2003, Bury 2001, Frank 1995, Kleinman 1988). I do not analyse the narrative *as* narrative, but rather as a more or less accurate and apt representation – which is also, of course, a partial and situated perspective – of a particular disease regime at two different moments in time. Extending Troy Duster's (1989) notion of the structural anecdote, I treat Larson's testimony as a *structural narrative*. In this case, the structure in question is the regime of breast cancer.

This is not a naive reading of Larson's testimony, however, because Clara's illness experience does not constitute the main source of evidence for the arguments and analysis that I develop. Following the extended case method (Burawoy 1991, 1998), I mobilise Larson's narrative to illustrate and illuminate a larger story about the impact of social movements on disease regimes and illness experience. I mobilise this larger story, in turn, to address weaknesses in the current state of theorising about illness experience (see Pierret 2003) and contribute to their reformulation. The evidence for this larger story is based upon original ethnographic and historical research and informed by existing scholarship.

In this chapter I situate Clara Larson's narrative within the San Francisco Bay Area field of social movements. My understanding of this field is based upon four years of ethnographic research in the San Francisco Bay Area, conducted between 1994 and 1998. This research included the observation of women's cancer support groups (a total of four groups, in four different organisational settings, for periods of time ranging from two months to two years) and participant observation in a range of locally-based social movement organisations, networks, projects, fundraisers, cultural events, educational forums, environmental protests, street theatre, public hearings, community-based early detection campaigns, conferences and symposia. This ethnographic research was supplemented by secondary historical research and more than 40 taped interviews and oral histories of current and former cancer patients, activists, educators, scientists, support group leaders and volunteers in the San Francisco Bay Area. In addition to these original sources of data, my analysis is informed by breast cancer narratives written by patients, survivors and activists; studies of breast cancer activism and the women's health movement; studies of breast cancer illness narratives and illness experiences; studies of breast cancer in popular culture; and historical research on early detection campaigns and the medical management of breast cancer[3].

Breast cancer in two regimes

The disease regime that Clara Larson faced when she was diagnosed with breast cancer in 1979 was one that emerged in the early part of the 20th century and held sway until the 1970s, when it gradually began to shift. By the time Clara Larson was diagnosed with breast cancer for the second time, a new regime of breast cancer had taken shape in the San Francisco Bay Area. This section explores those changes, as seen through the eyes of Clara Larson.

The first part of Larson's narrative illuminates some of the defining qualities of the earlier regime of breast cancer, even as it was beginning to change. These include the sovereign power of physicians (surgeons in particular); the isolation, normalisation and disempowerment of patients; the hegemony of gender normative and heteronormative assumptions about female embodiment, attractiveness and sexuality; the invisibility of women with breast cancer and 'mastectomees' in the public domain (despite the public disclosures of a handful of celebrities) and the absence of a group identity. This earlier regime was indeed rather totalising, but Larson's narrative reveals how her lesbian identity and feminist experiences and sensibilities provided her with the intellectual tools and the social and emotional resources to maintain a critical distance – a self-protective barrier of sorts – from the technologies of control and normalisation that she encountered.

The second part of Larson's narrative illuminates some of the defining qualities of the second, emergent regime. These include the dethroning of surgeons, the replacement of the surgeon-patient dyad with a web of relationships, the expansion of patients' access to medical information and their right to fully participate in medical decision-making; the creation of new social spaces, services and resources for women with breast cancer; the growing visibility of breast cancer patients and ex-patients in the public domain, the emergence of new collective identities and the development of a multi-stranded and multi-dimensional breast cancer movement.

Clara Larson in 1979: domination, isolation and the limits of resistance

In the early 1970s, when she was in her early thirties, Clara Larson followed the advice of her obstetrician/gynecologist and scheduled her first mammogram. Mammograms had been used as a diagnostic tool since the 1950s, but it was not until the 1970s that the National Cancer Institute (NCI) and the American Cancer Society (ACS) began to heavily promote the use of mammography as a breast cancer screening technology. Clara was part of the first wave of healthy, asymptomatic women to undergo routine mammographic screening, and she did so before the age and safety guidelines for mammographic screening were challenged and changed (though the debate rages on)[4]. Clara recalls that she began getting mammograms in the early 1970s:

> I know that now they say that for a woman under 50 it [a screening mammogram] should be every two years, but then it was every year. My doctor said 'this is something you need to do now, so go here and do this'. and so that's what I did.

In 1979 a routine mammogram revealed a suspicious lump in Clara's breast. Six weeks later she went into the hospital to have the lump biopsied. Clara entered the hospital expecting to emerge a few hours later with a clean bill of health. But things did not go as planned. As Clara recalled:

> I had the biopsy and I was in the recovery room because I had general anesthesia, that's what they did then, and this giant person loomed over me in his green outfit and he said, 'Well it's cancer! Do you want me to cut it off now or in a couple of days?'

Recalling this experience in vivid detail almost 20 years later, Clara said, 'so I allowed as how [so I told him that] I would like to wait a couple of days'. Shaking her head and laughing in outrage and disbelief she continued:

> But he was just gonna do it! Right then and there! And me explaining things to my kids, or making arrangements for them and my dog and cat – or whatever! It was totally unimportant [to him]. He just wanted to wheel me back in and cut my breast off! What an idiot! . . . He's actually still around. But I'll bet he can't get away with that anymore.

Clara was more fortunate than many others. At the time of her diagnosis, neither professional norms nor legal regulations required surgeons to separate the diagnosis of breast cancer from its surgical treatment, nor to inform their patients of alternatives (Montini 1997). This so-called 'one-step procedure' required patients to sign in advance a form authorising the surgeon to perform an immediate mastectomy if cancer were found, or believed to be found. Later that same year, the NIH held a Consensus Development Conference on the treatment of primary breast cancer and issued a series of findings, including the non-binding recommendation that surgeons discuss treatment alternatives with their patients and abandon the one-step procedure (NIH 1979). In 1980 California became the second state to pass breast cancer informed consent legislation. This legislation did not criminalise the one-step procedure, but it did characterise as 'unprofessional conduct' the failure of a physician 'to inform a patient being treated for any form of breast cancer of alternative, efficacious methods of treatment' (CDC 2000). Thus, instead of awakening to the voice of her surgeon informing her that she had breast cancer and asking whether she wanted him to 'cut it off' now or later, Clara could easily have awoken to the voice of her surgeon telling her that, while she was unconscious, he had diagnosed and treated her for breast cancer by removing her breast, her chest muscles and her lymph nodes. As callous as Clara's surgeon surely proved himself to be, he was actually on the progressive end of the spectrum on this issue.

Diagnosed with breast cancer at the age of 37, Clara went home to make hasty arrangements for the care of her four children, then returned to the hospital for surgery and underwent a radical mastectomy. After spending three or four days recovering in the hospital, she returned home in time to take her final exams and finish her first semester of graduate school. As Clara recalled:

> There was no process. No sensitivity to any feelings I might have about this. Or anything! It was very mechanical. . . . The medical establishment was horrible. Horrible. Horrible. Horrible. . . . It was just kind of like you were having your tonsils out. . . . I just don't remember any supportive medical personnel at all.

In addition to surgery, Clara had one appointment with a medical oncologist, who determined that adjuvant therapy was unnecessary. At her follow-up appointment with her surgeon, on the other hand, Clara was advised to undergo an additional, elective procedure:

> This was a time when I was visiting him myself [without her lover/partner Regina]. And he said, 'You know, you really need to have reconstructive surgery'. and I said, 'Why?' and he said, 'I have seen many a marriage founder on the shoals of a mastectomy'. and I thought, 'Okay. I'm gay. Now how do I explain this to a guy in a way that doesn't make it sound like my body's not important in this relationship . . . and I got so confused trying to figure out how I should respond to him . . . that I lost the opportunity. And I never did explain that to him.

Asked what it was that she had wanted to communicate to her surgeon almost 20 years earlier, Clara responded:

> I wanted him to know that I was gay, and that he shouldn't talk to me about heterosexual marriage. But I couldn't figure out how to do it without making it sound . . . I couldn't figure out how to give him the right message. I don't think he could have heard it anyway . . . If I were to explain it to him today I would say, 'This is my body and I see no reason to try to protect people from the fact that I have cancer. Had cancer. Whatever. That is their problem if they can't deal with it'. But at the time it did not occur to me [how] to explain that to him.

Reflecting later, Clara said:

> I can imagine if I had been straight that that really would have affected me. But I just thought it was weird! and I didn't know how to verbally respond to make myself understood by this goon. So I think it would have affected me. It would have hurt my feelings. It would have worried me. It would have scared me. If I had not been a lesbian . . . I probably would have killed myself or started drinking.

She added:

> My body was my body. And certainly I went through all the
> consciousness-raising groups in the seventies and . . . certainly, the
> women's movement and all that stuff that we were going through in the
> seventies gave me words and concepts to be able to understand how I
> felt about this stuff . . . And certainly if I hadn't been through all that
> stuff, I don't know that I would have been a lesbian. I'd probably still be
> married to Sally's [her daughter's] father. And I would have taken the stuff
> that that doctor said to me very seriously. And I would have been worried
> about it, because it certainly echoed the messages about femininity and
> womanhood that I'd learned growing up . . . And if I hadn't been freed
> from it by the women's movement, then I just would have . . . I wouldn't
> have questioned it . . . If you don't have the words to express how you feel,
> you're really kind of stuck with the feeling. And that's what I got out of
> those early years and it definitely . . . definitely created my response to the
> whole cancer experience.

Instead of internalising the sexism and heterosexism of her surgeon,
Clara's feminism and her lesbian identity provided her with the emotional,
experiential and intellectual resources to reject these male, heterocentric
assumptions about women's breasts, bodies, desires, pains, pleasures, preferences
and priorities.

From the healthcare system's point of view, Clara's rehabilitation was
simple and speedy. In the 1970s the only institutionalised form of rehabilitation
and support available to women with breast cancer was Reach to Recovery,
a programme adopted by the American Cancer Society in 1969 to provide support and practical advice to post-surgical mastectomy patients (Ross 1987: 161–
71). Reach to Recovery was designed to appease the concerns of surgeons,
many of whom initially viewed the programme with a mixture of scepticism
and suspicion (1987: 167–8). Access to patients was controlled by physicians, and Reach to Recovery volunteers were prohibited from expressing their
opinions or offering advice about physicians, treatments or medical concerns
(1987: 167–8).

The programme was organised so that a Reach to Recovery volunteer, always
a former breast cancer patient, would visit the new 'mastectomee' shortly after
surgery, either in the hospital or, less desirably, in her home. The Reach to
Recovery volunteer would teach her temporary charge how to perform therapeutic exercises, which were designed to aid in her physical recovery, and
how to hide the evidence of her surgery with a breast prosthesis, which was
designed to aid in her psychological recovery. Dr. Markel, a strong supporter
of the programme in the 1970s, offered the following analysis:

> I think the big bang in Reach to Recovery is when the patient in the bed
> looks up and a woman comes through the door. (And we insist [that she]

wear a tight fitting gown so that both breasts show and her hair is all combed.) We think we've made it then at that point. She [the patient] looks up. You are a Reach to Recovery volunteer and you've had a mastectomy. If something clicks here, then all the rest of it is not terribly important, because then she wants to get well (quoted in Breslow 1979: 460).

Reach to Recovery reflected, responded to and reinforced the relationship between women's social status and gender identity on the one hand, and their physical attractiveness and 'breasted experience' (Young 1990) on the other. The goal of the programme was for the post-surgery patient to re-enter her former life and become again the person she was before she was diagnosed and treated for breast cancer. The goal of the programme was *not* to create social networks and a supportive community, but to facilitate a quick transition back to normality.

In *Breast Cancer: A Personal History and Investigative Report* (1975), Rose Kushner wrote about the difficulties she encountered in her efforts to gather information on women treated for breast cancer. Wanting to contact women who were not immediately 'post-op', Kushner turned to the American Cancer Society and its Reach to Recovery programme for help. The ACS was unable to assist, however, because the Reach to Recovery programme did not keep records or maintain contact with the women who had been visited by their volunteers. Kushner described a conversation she had had with a representative of the ACS concerning this issue. The representative explained to Kushner:

'We didn't want Reach to Recovery to become a crutch . . . After all, the whole point of Reach to Recovery is to convince women they do not have a disabling handicap. We talked about having a mastectomy club, like the various ostomy clubs and laryngectomy clubs. But that would have defeated our whole purpose. Having a mastectomy is not a handicap, and even the worst of scars can be hidden by a well-fitting prosthesis and the right clothing. We decided we would help the patient for just a few weeks, and then leave her to her own psychological recovery' (Kushner 1975: 211).

For many women, being visited by a Reach to Recovery volunteer was a welcome experience. It provided them with their only link to the mastectomy underground. For Clara, however, this experience was one of alienation instead of sisterhood:

I felt sorry for her. I mean, she meant well. She really meant well. But, you know, she wanted to tell me all about prostheses and how you could dress to minimize looking like you'd had a mastectomy and . . . it was not what I needed. I got rid of her as soon as I could.

Later, looking back on her first brush with breast cancer, Clara shared an interesting insight about the impact of breast cancer on her relationship to heteronormative standards of beauty. She explained that although being diagnosed with a life-threatening disease had been terrifying, and losing her breast had been traumatic, not everything about the experience was negative:

> One of the interesting things about having cancer is that it's not all bad. In some ways it's very freeing. . . . One of the epiphanies the first time was that, like all young American girls, I mean, I grew up in the forties and fifties . . . I was oppressed by the idea that I had to be beautiful and I had to look like a Playboy centerfold, which I never did. I was never beautiful. I never looked like that. I never *could* have looked like that! It would have been impossible. And it tortured me. And having cancer really liberated me from that. It was like, 'Okay, I only have one breast now so I can't possibly compete!' And it was extremely freeing! I didn't have to try anymore! I didn't have to worry about it. I was out of the running . . . That part was really cool. I loved that.

Clara never opted for reconstructive surgery and she neither acquired nor wore a prosthesis. She continued wearing her same clothing, tight tank-tops and T-shirts. She continued taking her children to the public swimming pool wearing her old bikini. 'I was very exhibitionist about it', she said, 'especially at the beginning . . . and people were shocked!'.

Clara 'went on' with her life, as she put it, without hiding the visible signs of her cancer history. But she was forced to come to terms with this history and to make sense of it without the benefit of other women who shared her experience. As Clara recalled:

> In 1979 people just wanted you to have surgery and they didn't want to talk about it . . . You were in and out of the hospital and that was that! There was no social workers, no support groups . . . the closest thing to that was the Reach to Recovery lady and that was awful . . . and that was all there was. There wasn't anybody! I didn't know a single soul! and . . . um . . . that would have been nice, if I'd known other people. Yup. That would have been nice. Because . . . my partner certainly didn't understand it. I mean, nobody understands this experience unless they've gone through it. They just really don't . . . But I had no idea how to get ahold of people. And the Women's Cancer Resource Center [a feminist community cancer centre in Berkeley] didn't exist. It wasn't there. And there were no resources that I knew of.

Thus, except for follow-up appointments, Clara was officially 'done' with breast cancer when she recovered from surgery. Summarising the environment for women with breast cancer in the late 1970s, Clara said:

> People didn't talk about it then. And I think that's probably the most global thing that I can say about having breast cancer in 1979. People. Didn't. Talk. About it. Period.

Although she was part of the first wave of women who were mammographically screened for breast cancer, Clara knew almost nothing about the disease either before or after her diagnosis. Scientific studies and medical information were not readily available and breast cancer patients, even middle class graduate students, had not yet become lay-experts. In theory, Clara could have gone to a medical library and conducted her own research, but this was not something that it occurred to her to do. This was not something that patients typically did. This was true despite the fact that Clara was active in the women's movement, despite the fact that she possessed a healthy distrust of the medical establishment, and despite the fact that her lover/partner, Regina, was a physician. Even if medical information had been accessible, the treatment options available to her were negligible, the room for manoeuvring almost non-existent.

Clara was unusual in that she forced open the space of participation and created an alternative path. She chose not to hide the evidence of her mastectomy. She refused, as she put it 'to protect people from seeing this'. Her visibility to others, however, did not make others visible to her. Clara explained that she used to walk down the street after she had learned, much to her surprise, that one in 13 women (now one in seven) could expect to meet a similar fate. She remembers looking in vain for those invisible one-in-13 women and wondering who and where they were. She thought of her friends and all the women she knew. She wondered how many of them would get breast cancer – and she wondered, as she said, 'how many of them already had'. In 1979 Clara's act of refusal was a symbolic gesture without a language, disembedded from the context and community necessary to recognise and respond to it. Although Clara struggled against the limits of this disease regime, those limits were finite and rigid. Feminism, women's liberation and a lesbian identity could take her only so far. They could change her relationship to the regime of breast cancer and they could buffer her against its sharper edges, but they could not, or rather, they had not yet, thoroughly transformed the practices of this regime.

Clara Larson in 1997: new social relations, solidarities and subjectivities

In 1997 Clara was diagnosed with metastatic breast cancer when she sought medical treatment for a back injury. In the end, rumours of a cure proved to be greatly exaggerated, as they did for so many women who were optimistially but prematurely pronounced 'cured'. Prognostically speaking, Clara's second diagnosis was much worse than her first. By 1997 her original breast cancer had metastasised to her vertebrae, her hip and her lungs.

This time round, Clara turned to a variety of sources of information and was gratified by what she found:

> The Internet was really helpful. And then you've got the 1-800-4CANCER [the NCI cancer information number]. And I know a lot more people who've had cancer. And . . . there's the cancer center, and the cancer center is just so full of people who are helpful and tell you things, and my doctor is incredibly helpful and supportive. I mean, everybody's just really nice.

Clara used the web to research the chemotherapeutic drugs she was given and she checked out the breast cancer chat rooms and bulletin boards. She received gifts of books from family and friends. Her son, for example, presented her with a copy of *Cancer in Two Voices* (1991), an illness narrative written by a lesbian couple, Sandra Butler and Barbara Rosenblum, chronicling their life together, and Rosenblum's illness and death from breast cancer. Another friend gave her a copy of *Dr. Susan Love's Breast Book* (1995). A well-known breast cancer surgeon, as well as a feminist, a lesbian and a breast cancer activist, Love's book was wildly popular among women diagnosed with breast cancer.

But it was not just that access to information had expanded, the whole environment of healthcare delivery had changed. Contrasting the breast cancer regime of 1997 with that of 1979, Clara said:

> I just don't remember any supportive medical personnel at all [in 1979]. In contrast to what I'm going through now, where, you know, I'm in an HMO [Health Management Organisation], and healthcare is [supposed to be] so terrible and so seemingly unavailable . . . but the medical people have just been fabulous this time around. They're just wonderful. And that just didn't happen before.

Not only were the hospital staff and healthcare professionals helpful and supportive, but the sexism and heterosexism that infused her first encounter with the regime of breast cancer had been replaced (at least in the Berkeley hospital where Clara was treated) by a lesbian and feminist-friendly staff whose own views of breast cancer had been influenced by the breast cancer movement. As Clara said:

> A lot of these women are feminists, a lot of these women are lesbians. And people have a political consciousness about the whole cancer thing.

She continued:

> I mean, in Berkeley it is so okay to be gay – it's just totally okay. [It's] totally accepted. Now. Not before. And people have been fabulous with Susan [her new lover]. They treat her as my partner. They give her all

the respect that they would give a heterosexual partner . . . One woman, she wasn't a nurse, she was a pharmacist or something, and she came into my room to ask me about something and she said, 'well you're a lesbian aren't you?' and I thought, 'Whoa! What an assumption! What a turn around!' And gradually they all [the lesbian healthcare workers] came out to me. It was great. . . . It was fabulous. I loved it.

What a contrast to Clara's first experience of breast cancer! In 1979 Clara's lesbian identity was either invisible or ignored by her surgeon, who did not appear to think twice about his assumptions. Now the presumptuousness ran in the opposite direction – but in a way that delighted Clara and made her feel seen, recognised and accepted.

Not only had the social and cultural environment of cancer care changed, but so too had the organisation and delivery of services. Instead of feeling isolated and powerless, as she had in 1979, Clara felt like the captain of a well-functioning team dedicated to aiding and assisting her treatment and recovery. She gave a long list of the individuals who she viewed as members of her team:

Well certainly there's my oncologist. Then there's my regular general practitioner. There's my acupuncturist. There's my chiropractor. Also, my acupuncturist is an herbalist. And then there's other people that have been helpful in this process. . . . A couples counselor . . . and I would also put on the list my hair cutter [who shaved her head when she started losing her hair and continued shaving it during chemotherapy] . . . and I would also put my housecleaner on that list because I'm not supposed to get anywhere near dust [due to her compromised immune system]. And so the list just goes on and on and on and I feel like all those people have really contributed to solving the problem.

In addition to revealing the tremendous impact of alternative health movements on the Bay Area regime of breast cancer, this passage reveals one of the ways in which, increasingly, the experiences of illness available to women diagnosed with breast cancer were being shaped by class distinctions. In the earlier regime of breast cancer there was more of a 'one size fits all' approach to the diagnosis and treatment of disease, and treatment itself, especially for women diagnosed with early stage breast cancer, was fairly simple (albeit radical) and straightforward – amputation of the breast. With minimal options, alternatives and amenities available to women diagnosed with breast cancer, the social, cultural and economic capital (see Bourdieu 1986) possessed by individual patients was less consequential. There were simply fewer investment opportunities – fewer ways of converting these various forms of capital into better treatment outcomes and illness experiences. In contrast, between April 1997 (her second diagnosis) and January 1998 (when she was interviewed), Clara estimated that she spent $6,000 of her own money on alternative and complementary treatments and services not covered by her HMO. Beyond that, the treatment that she received, a stem cell transplant, was an expensive and experimental procedure to which few women with breast cancer had access. Ironically, despite the popular backlash against a healthcare system increasingly organised around the logic of market mechanisms (see Scott *et al.* 2000 for an institutional analysis of these transformations in the Bay Area), certain dimensions of the regime of breast cancer had improved for middle class patients. By 1997 middle class breast cancer patients with health insurance in the San Francisco Bay Area had become savvy consumers, forcing medical facilities to compete for this ever-expanding market. The number of 'women's health' and 'breast health' centres grew during the 1990s, along with special resources, support groups and other amenities. These improvements did not benefit all patients equally, however, and almost certainly exacerbated existing inequalities (see especially Shaffer 2000), but they did contribute in positive ways to the illness experience of medically-empowered patients.

The cancer centre where Clara received her treatment offered free patient education workshops and cancer support groups. These were organised according to various criteria: type of cancer, stage of cancer, age, sex, etc. There were drop-in groups, ongoing groups and coed groups for people with metastatic disease. If Clara had wanted to avoid medical settings (as many cancer patients do), there were free support groups and educational forums in alternative settings. Just down the street, the Women's Cancer Resource Center (WCRC) offered a series of support groups, including one for lesbians with cancer. They also offered a variety of practical services to women with cancer, including a medical library, research assistance, patients' evaluations of local physicians, phone access to women willing to share their treatment experiences and one-on-one assistance with transportation, shopping, cleaning and other errands and activities. Further down the road, the Charlotte Maxwell Complementary Clinic provided free complementary and alternative cancer therapies (massage, acupuncture, Chinese herbs, meditation, etc.) and organic fruits and vegetables to low-income women with cancer.

Clara attended a series of workshops for cancer patients who, like her, were contemplating undergoing a stem cell transplant. These workshops provided Clara with an opportunity to establish relationships with other, similarly-positioned patients and put her in touch with additional resources, support and information. Certainly, Clara did not access all, or even a significant portion of the resources available to her, but their existence, and her awareness of their existence, nonetheless shaped her illness experience by changing what had been (in 1979) an individualised experience of isolation and alienation into a shared experience of support and solidarity.

Even Clara's son benefited from the new openness about breast cancer. Clara related a story about her son, who ran into an old friend of his from high school. According to Clara, her son's friend asked, innocently enough,

'How's your mother?' – and her son responded that his mother had been diagnosed with cancer. His friend replied 'Mine too! What kind of cancer does your mom have?' 'Breast cancer', her son explained. His friend once again responded 'Mine too!' Clara smiled and said, 'This never would have happened when I was growing up! We never would have had a conversation like that about our mothers in the 1950s'. Instead of hiding their mother's stigmatising illnesses and suffering alone and in silence, these two young men were able to bond over their shared experience, support one another and renew their friendship.

But even for a white, middle class, lesbian feminist living in Berkeley, California the new regime of breast cancer was not a disease utopia. Clara, for example, did not particularly like the Women's Cancer Resource Center. As she explained:

> They reminded me of . . . in the seventies all the lesbians that I knew
> . . . were downwardly mobile . . . and there was a certain way that you
> were supposed to be . . . and I had way too many kids to be politically
> correct, and I also lived a very middle class lifestyle . . . and there were
> a lot of people that were very critical of me because I wasn't the right
> kind of lesbian. And that's the same feeling that I had when I walked into
> WCRC. And I'm sure that this is not everybody's experience, but it was
> my experience . . . and that probably had a lot to do with my resentment
> with all the people who basically just discounted me in the seventies
> because I wasn't a politically correct lesbian. I guess it [Clara's negative
> reaction] probably just hooked into that.

Although WCRC was a feminist and lesbian-friendly organisation, Clara did not respond positively to its organisational culture because it evoked painful memories of rejection, which in turn inspired feelings of anger and resentment. She felt rejected not by WCRC per se, but by the lesbian feminist community with which she associated it, a community that, 20 years ago, had rejected her, she believed, for being too mainstream, too middle class and too motherly.

This aspect of Clara's illness experience is a powerful reminder of two things. First, it reminds us of the importance of cultural differences, even within groups we assume are relatively homogenous. In this case, differences in class culture and political culture separated Clara from an organisation for which one might reasonably have expected her to feel a fair amount of enthusiasm. Furthermore, giving an ironic twist to sociological assumptions about class-based exclusions, Clara felt rejected not for being too poor, but for being too middleclass. Second, it reminds us that disease regimes shape, rather than determine, illness experience. The development of lesbian and feminist cancer organisations created new social spaces, solidarities and subjectivities, vastly expanding the kinds of illness experiences available within the second regime of breast cancer. But individual experiences, memories, personalities and perspectives also shape illness experience.

Just as Clara's feminist politics and lesbian identity served as resources during her first encounter with the regime of breast cancer, painful memories of rejection by the lesbian community created barriers to fully accessing the resources for women with cancer later provided by the lesbian community.

Social movements in the Bay Area also changed the way in which the issue of breast cancer was publicly framed and understood. Environmental activism was a key focus of the breast cancer movement in the San Francisco Bay Area. By 1998 this particular orientation had crept into Clara Larson's own cognitive framework and political sensibilities. No longer did she view breast cancer solely through the lens of gender and sexuality. She now viewed breast cancer as an environmental disease and an issue of corporate profits and pollution. As Clara explained:

> In those days [after her first diagnosis], I thought it [wearing breast prostheses] was to protect men from seeing that there were women walking around with one tit. And now I think it's because . . . the increase in cancer, I believe, is environmental. And people need to be protected from us so that they don't realize what an epidemic this is, especially here in the Bay Area, and start questioning some of the people who are polluting the environment, polluting the bay. Because that's big corporate money. And they don't want people to think about it. That's also why they focus on detection instead of prevention.

Clara indicated that she had arrived at this analysis 'probably in the last five years, when I started hearing the statistics that breast cancer is so much more prevalent in the Bay Area than anywhere else in the country'. The wide circulation and politicisation of these statistics, framed as evidence of environmental influences, was the handiwork of the feminist cancer and environmental justice movements (see Klawiter 2003). Clara's understanding of breast cancer was thus shaped by environmental breast cancer activism even though she was not active in this, or any other, social movement.

In fact, Clara's lack of involvement was the source of some remorse. She explained that when breast cancer activism started developing in the Bay Area in the late 1980s and early 1990s, a lot of her friends assumed that she would love to get involved. But, as Clara said, 'I just didn't want to'. 'For me', Clara explained, 'my cancer experience was really . . . awful and it was something that I wanted to leave behind. I didn't feel like going up there and being part of all that. I would have rather volunteered at the SPCA [Society for the Prevention of Cruelty to Animals] or something'. Since her second diagnosis, Clara had been feeling a growing sense of moral obligation to get involved in the breast cancer movement: 'I think I should get involved', she said, 'but I bet that I won't'. She continued:

> I think that something has to be done about it and it's important to push for more money for research, and it's important to be part of the

movement to expose the environmental hazards and all that kind of stuff. That's important work to be done . . . but I probably won't do it, because when this is over, I'm gonna want to shut it out of my life again.

Larson's desire to keep her distance was not in the least bit unusual or difficult to comprehend. After all, most people, given the choice, would prefer to put the experience of cancer behind them. The difference is that, in 1979, Clara looked for political community but was unable to find it. In 1998, she felt called upon to justify her lack of political involvement.

Despite her reticence, Clara discovered that she could witness the political face of breast cancer from within the privacy of her own living room. That summer, while reclining on her couch and recovering from a stem-cell transplant with high-dosage chemotherapy, Clara watched as lesbian, feminist and environmental cancer activists marched in San Francisco's annual lesbian-gay-bisexual-transgender pride parade. One-breasted, two-breasted and bare-breasted women marched at the front of the parade, carrying the official parade banner. That year, as the banner indicated, the parade was officially dedicated 'To Our Sisters with Cancer'. Groups from the Women's Cancer Resource Center, Charlotte Maxwell Complementary Clinic, Lyon-Martin Women's Health Services, Breast Cancer Action and the Toxic Links Coalition trailed behind. A handful of women covered with colourful, plastic, mini-breast prostheses handed out flyers and threw Frisbees advertising free mammograms for low-income women. Behind them, a couple of dozen women and several men carried cardboard gravestones emblazoned with the names of women, both famous and obscure, who had died of breast cancer. Bringing up the rear was a trolley car full of women who, as their banner indicated, were 'living with cancer'. This time around, instead of 'taking it to the streets' all alone and finding neither camaraderie nor political community, Clara watched comfortably from her couch as images of breast cancer activists taking over the streets of San Francisco were beamed back into her living room.

Conclusions

Although Clara Larson was, and is, a truly exceptional individual, what she encountered and endured when she was diagnosed with breast cancer in the late 1970s was neither exceptional nor extreme. In the first regime, her experience of breast cancer was relentlessly individualised. She looked for a sisterhood of survivors but never found one. She engaged in acts of civil disobedience but remained isolated. Surgeons were the undisputed sovereigns within the medical setting, and structurally speaking, the only role available to women with breast cancer was that of the duly compliant patient. Almost inevitably, the power inequalities structured into the physician-patient relationship were deepened by the gender-inequalities between male surgeons and female patients. Even an atypical patient like Clara, who had been involved in consciousness-raising, women's liberation and lesbian feminism (and whose partner was a physician) found the power dynamics and disparities overwhelming. The women's movement and lesbian feminism provided her with the intellectual, social and emotional resources to maintain a critical distance from some of the technologies of normalisation, but there were practical limits to her resistance, and those limits were established by the regime of breast cancer.

By 1997, however, a new regime of breast cancer had emerged in the San Francisco Bay Area. Not only had the clinical contours of disease changed, but the public face of breast cancer had undergone a remarkable transformation. Clara was treated in a feminist and lesbian-friendly cancer centre. She decided between medical alternatives, attended patient-education workshops, participated in her treatment as a member of a 'healthcare team' that consisted of a range of healthcare professionals – both regular and alternative – and an assortment of support personnel. Books by lesbian feminist surgeons and patients appeared in her hands. Support groups, medical information and practical resources for women with breast cancer were freely available. Women with breast cancer had become a visible presence in the public domain and breast cancer survivors were now heralded as heroes rather than pitied as victims. Breast cancer had been politicised along multiple dimensions and reframed, among other things, as a feminist issue and an environmental disease. And the gay pride parade, which was dedicated to women with cancer, marched right into her living room.

The contrast between the first and second regimes of breast cancer was dramatic. In the earlier regime of practices, Clara attempted to take breast cancer to the streets by making visible its inscription on her body. But she did so alone, and her impact was necessarily limited. Instead of sisterhood and solidarity, she crashed into the rigid structure of stigma, isolation and invisibility – the architecture of the closet. The second time she was diagnosed with breast cancer Clara maintained her distance from the social movements engaged in breast cancer activism. They changed her experience of illness nonetheless, because they radically transformed the regime of practices through which her experience of breast cancer was constituted.

So what does this study contribute to our understanding of the structural shaping of illness experience? How does it address gaps in our scholarship and weaknesses in our theorising? It does so in four respects. First, it offers the concept of disease regime. Conceptualising disease as a regime of practices allows us to analyse structures as practices, and enhances our ability to historicise and contextualise the structural shaping of illness experience. If there were ever a time when the social construction of disease and the social structuring of illness could be understood by limiting one's focus to the institutions of science and medicine, and the social relations of class, race, gender, etc., that time has surely passed. We need frameworks that recognise the multiplicity of practices and institutions shaping the social structuring of disease and illness experience; we need frameworks that recognise the multiplicity of arenas in which these practices are played out and contested. Second, this study demonstrates the value of incorporating social movements more fully into the study of illness experience. Social movements are not the only source of change, of course, but they are an increasingly important one – and one that has been undertheorised thus far in the scholarship on illness experience. At the same time, scholarship on health and illness-related social movements tends to focus on their success in legislative and policy-making arenas. This study shifts the focus to what, after all, constitutes one of the most important measures of success: their impact on the lived experience of so-called 'free riders' and non-participants. Third, this study proposes that social movements change illness experience in two ways: by changing the sufferer's relationship to the regime of practices, and by changing the actual practices of the disease regime. Even social movements that do not specifically target disease regimes can have an impact on the illness experiences of individuals, but the impact is necessarily limited if they do not change the experiences of illness that disease regimes make available. Finally, this study underscores the significance of gender and sexuality to the analysis of illness experience, demonstrating how gender and sexuality are constituted within disease regimes and challenged by social movements.

Acknowledgements

For their insight, comments and suggestions on earlier drafts of this chapter, I am grateful to Phil Brown, Stephen Zavestoski, Mike Allen and the editor and anonymous reviewers of *Sociology of Health and Illness*.

Notes

1 Corporate contributions to the 'beautification' of breast cancer are discussed in greater length elsewhere (Klawiter 1999b). See Samantha King (2001) for an exceptionally thoughtful analysis of the relationship between breast cancer-related corporate philanthropy, cause-related marketing and new forms of citizenship. See also Suein L. Hwang (1993), Lisa Belkin (1996), Debra Goldman (1997), Sandy M. Fernandez (1998, 1999), Mary Ann Swissler (2002), and Breast Cancer Action's 'Think Before You Pink' campaign (*http://www.thinkbeforeyoupink.org*).
2 There is significant overlap between social movements and what I am referring to as the 'non-establishment approaches of medically marginalised communities'. See, for example, David Hess (2003) and Gerald E. Markle, James C. Petersen and Morton O. Wagenfeld (1978).
3 My analysis is informed by breast cancer narratives written by patients, survivors and activists (Kushner 1977a, 1977b, 1986, Lorde 1980, Winnow 1989, 1991, Brady 1991, Butler and Rosenbeum 1991, Stocker 1991, 1993, Mayer 1993, Batt 1994, Dunnavant 1995, Kahane 1995, Altman 1996, Orenstein 1997, Midddlebrook 1997); studies of breast cancer activism (Montini and Ruzek 1989, Montini and Slobin 1991, Dickerson 1996, Montini 1996, 1997, Taylor and Van Willigen 1996, Anglin

1997, Densham 1997, Kaufert 1998, Leopold 1999, Brenner 2000, Fishman 2000, Weisman 2000, King 2001, Casamayou 2001, McCormick *et al.* 2003, Brown *et al.* 2004, Zavestoski *et al.* in press) and the women's health movement (Ruzek 1978, Norsigian 1996, Weisman 1998); studies of breast cancer illness narratives and illness experiences (Hawkins 1993, Mathews, Lanin, and Mitchell 1994, Leopold 1999, Rosenbaum and Roos 2000, Potts 2000, Kasper 2000); studies of breast cancer in popular culture (Clarke 1992, Lupton 1994, Yadlon 1997, Yalom 1997, Lantz and Booth 1998, Leopold 1999, Lerner 2001, Marino 1999, Fosket 2000, Saywell 2000, Brown *et al.* 2001); and historical research on early detection campaigns and the medical management of breast cancer (Breslow 1979, Ross 1987, Patterson 1987, Fisher 1985, 1999, Balshem 1993, Cartwright 1995, Gardner 1999, Leopold 1999, Lerner 2000, 2001, Aronowitz 2001).

4   The NCI and the ACS began promoting mammographic screening for breast cancer in the early 1970s, through the Breast Cancer Early Detection Demonstration Project. The BCDDP provoked a number of controversies about the safety, wisdom and effectiveness of mammographic screening that, after 20 more years of clinical trials and meta-analyses, have only become more complicated (see Bailer 1976, Rennie 1977, Breslow 1979, Baker 1982, Ross 1987, Skrabanek 1989, Kaufert 1996, Linden 1998, Olsen and Gotzsche 2001, Sherman 2002, Joyce 2003, Stein 2004).

References

Altman, R. (1996) *Waking Up, Fighting Back: The Politics of Breast Cancer*. New York: Little, Brown, and Company.

Anglin, M.K. (1997) Working from the inside out: implications of breast cancer activism for biomedical policies and practices, *Social Science and Medicine*, 44, 9, 1403–15.

Armstrong, D. (1993) Public health spaces and the fabrication of identity, *Sociology*, 27, 3, 393–410.

Armstrong, D. (1995) The rise of surveillance medicine, *Sociology of Health and Illness*, 17, 3, 393–404.

Aronowitz, R. (2001) Do not delay: breast cancer and time, 1900–1970, *The Milbank Quarterly*, 79, 3, 355–86.

Bailar III, J.C. (1976) Mammography: a contrary view, *Annals of Internal Medicine*, 84, 77–84.

Baker, L.H. (1982) Breast cancer detection demonstration project: five-year summary report, *CA-A Cancer Journal for Clinicians*, 32, 194–227.

Balshem, M. (1993) *Cancer in the Community: Class and Medical Authority*. Washington, D.C.: Smithsonian Institution Press.

Batt, S. (1994) *Patient No More: The Politics of Breast Cancer*. Charlottetown: Canada: Gynergy Books.

Belkin, L. (1996) How breast cancer became this year's hottest charity, *New York Times Magazine*, 22 December.

Bourdieu, P. (1986) The Forms of Capital. In Richardson, J. (ed.) *Handbook of Theory and Research for the Sociology of Education*. New York: Greenwood Press.

Brady, J. (1991) (ed) *1 in 3: Women with Cancer Confront an Epidemic*. San Francisco: Cleis Press.

Brenner, B. (2000) Sister Support: Women Create a Breast Cancer Movement. In Kasper, A.S. and Ferguson, S.J. (eds) *Breast Cancer: Society Shapes an Epidemic*. New York: St. Martin's Press.

Breslow, L. (1979) *A History of Cancer Control in the United States with Emphasis on the Period 1946–1971*. Department of Health, Education & Welfare.

Brown, P. and Ferguson, F.I.T. (1995) Making a big stink: women's work, women's relationships, and toxic waste activism, *Gender and Society*, 9, 2, 145–72.

Brown, P., Zavestoski, S., McCormick, S., Mandelbaum, J. and Luebke, T. (2001) Print media coverage of environmental causation of breast cancer, *Sociology of Health and Illness*, 23, 6, 747–76.

Brown, P., Zavestoski, S., McCormick, S., Mayer, B., Morello-Frosch, R. and Gasior, R. (2004) Embodied health movements: uncharted territory in social movement research, *Sociology of Health and Illness*, 26, 1–31.

Bunton, R. and Burrows, R. (1995) Consumption and health in the 'epidemiological' clinic of late modern medicine. In Burrows, R., Nettleton, S. and Bunton, R. (eds) *The Sociology of Health Promotion: Critical Analyses of Consumption, Lifestyle and Risk*. London: Routledge.

Bunton, R. and Petersen, A. (1997) Introduction: Foucault's medicine. In Petersen, A. and Bunton, R. (eds) *Foucault: Health and Medicine*. London: Routledge.

Burawoy, M. (1991) Introduction. In Burawoy, M., Burbon, A., Ferguson, A.A. *et al.* (eds) *Ethnography Unbound: Power and Resistance in the Modern Metropolis*. Berkeley: University of California Press.

Burawoy, M. (1998) The extended case method, *Sociological Theory*, 16, 1, 4–33.

Burrows, R., Nettleton, S. and Bunton, R. (1995) Sociology and health promotion: health, risk and consumption under later modernism. In Burrows, R., Nettleton, S. and Bunton, R. (eds) *The Sociology of Health Promotion: Critical Analyses of Consumption, Lifestyle and Risk*. London: Routledge.

Bury, M. (2001) Illness narratives: fact or fiction? *Sociology of Health & Illness*, 23, 3, 263–85.

Butler, S. and Rosenblum, B. (1991) *Cancer in Two Voices*. San Francisco: Spinsters Book Company.

Cartwright, L. (1995) *Screening the Body: Tracing Medicine's Visual Culture*. Minneapolis: University of Minnesota Press.

Casamayou, M.H. (2001) *The Politics of Breast Cancer*. Washington D.C.: Georgetown University Press.

Castel, R. (1991) From Dangerousness to Risk. In Burchell, G., Gordon, C. and Miller, P. (eds) *The Foucault Effect: Studies in Governmentality*. Chicago: The University of Chicago Press.

Centers for Disease Control and Prevention (CDC) (2000) State Laws Relating to Breast Cancer: Legislative Summary January 1949 to May 2000. U.S. Department of Health and Human Services.

Clarke, J.N. (1992) Cancer, heat disease and AIDS: what do the media tell us about these diseases? *Health Communication*, 4, 2, 105–20.

Collins, P.H. (1999) Learning From the Outsider Within. In Hesse-Biber, S., Gilmartin, C. and Lydenberg, R. (eds) *Feminist Approaches to Theory and Methodology*. New York: Oxford University Press.

Connell, R.W. (1987) *Gender and Power*. Stanford: Stanford University Press.

Crossley, N. (1998) Transforming the mental health field, *Sociology of Health and Illness*, 20, 4, 458–88.

Crossley, N. (2003) The Field of Psychiatric Contention in the UK, 1960–2000. Paper presented at workshop, *Patient Organized Movements*, in Gotenborg, Sweden, 7–9 June.

Densham, A. (1997) The Marginalized Uses of Power and Identity: Lesbians' Participation in Breast Cancer and AIDS Activism. In Cohen, C.J., Jones, K.B. and Tronto, J.C. (eds) *Women Transforming Politics: An Alternative Reader*. New York: New York University Press.

Dickersin, K. and Schnaper, L. (1996) Reinventing Medical Research. In Moss, K.L. (ed) *Man-Made Medicine: Women's Health, Public Policy, and Reform*. Durham, NC: Duke University Press.

Doyal, L. (1995) *What Makes Women Sick: Gender and the Political Economy of Health*. New Brunswick: Rutgers University Press.

Dunnavant, S. (1995) *Celebrating Life: African American Women Speak Out About Breast Cancer*. Dallas: USFI, Inc.

Duster, T. (1989) The structural anecdote in social analysis, *Annual Meeting of the American Sociological Association*, San Francisco.

Fernandez, S.M. (1998) Pretty in pink, *Mamm: Women, Cancer and Community*, June/July.

Fernandez, S.M. (1999) Mamm's guide to breast cancer corporate bucks, *Mamm: Women, Cancer and Community*, 2, December/January, 32.

Ferraro, S. (1993) You can't look away anymore: the anguished politics of breast cancer, *New York Times Magazine*, 15 August, 1993.

Ferree, M.M. and Martin, P.Y. (1995) *Feminist Organizations: Harvest of the New Women's Movement*. Philadelphia: Temple University Press.

Ferree, M.M. and Roth, S. (1998) Gender, class, and the interaction between social movements: a strike of West Berlin day care workers, *Gender and Society*, 12, 626–48.

Fisher, B. (1985) The revolution of breast cancer surgery: science or anecdotation? *World Journal of Sugery*, 9, 655–66.

Fisher, B. (1999) From Halsted to prevention and beyond: advances in the management of breast cancer during the twentieth century, *European Journal of Cancer*, 35, 14, 1963–73.

Fishman, J. (2000) Assessing Breast Cancer: Risk, Science and Environmental Activism in an 'At Risk' Community. In Potts, L. (ed) *Ideologies of Breast Cancer: Feminist Perspectives*. New York: St. Martin's Press.

Fonow, M.M. (1998) Protest engendered: the participation of women steelworkers in the Wheeling-Pittsburgh steel strike of 1985, *Gender and Society*, 12, 710–28.

Fosket, J., Lafia, C. and Kanan, A. (2000) Breast Cancer in Popular Women's Magazines from 1913 to 1996. In Ferguson, S.J. and Kasper, A.S. (eds) *Breast Cancer: The Social Construction of Illess*. New York: St. Martin's Press.

Foucault, M. (1965) *Madness and Civilization*. London: Tavistock.

Foucault, M. (1973) *The Birth of the Clinic: An Archaeology of Medical Perception*. New York: Vintage Books.

Foucault, M. (1978) *History of Sexuality*, volume 1. New York: Pantheon Books.

Foucault, M. (1979) *Discipline and Punish: The Birth of the Prison*. New York: Vintage Books.

Foucault, M. (1980) The Politics of Health in the Eighteenth Century. In Gordon, C. (ed) *Power/Knowledge: Selected Interviews and Other Writings 1972–1977*. New York: Pantheon Books.

Foucault, M. (1987) Questions of Method: An Interview with Michel Foucault. In Baynes, K., Bohman, J. and McCarty, T. (eds) *After Philosophy – End or Transformation?* Boston: MIT Press.

Frank, A.W. (1995) *The Wounded Storyteller: Body, Illness, and Ethics.* Chicago: The University of Chicago Press.

Gamson, J. (1997) Messages of exclusion: gender, movements, and symbolic boundaries, *Gender and Society*, 11, 178–99.

Gardner, K.E. (1999) By women, for women, with women: a history of female cancer awareness efforts, 1913–1970s. Ph.D. Dissertation, Department of History: University of Cincinnati.

Goldman, D. (1997) Illness as Metaphor, *AdWeek*, 3 November, 70.

Hawkins, A. (1993) *Reconstructing Illness: Studies in Pathography.* West Lafayette, IN: Purtue University Press.

Hess, D.J. (2003) CAM Cancer Therapies in Twentieth-Century North America: The Emergence and Growth of a Social Movement. In Johnston, R.D. (ed) *The Politics of Healing: A History of Alternative Therapies in Twentieth-Century North America.* New York: Routledge.

Hwang, S.L. (1993) Linking products to breast cancer fight helps firms bond with their customers, *Wall Street Journal.*

Joyce, K. (2003) Legitimacy in Contemporary Medicine: The Not-So Difficult Integration of Controversial Technologies. *Annual Meeting of the American Sociological Association*, Atlanta.

Kahane, D.H. (ed) (1995) *No Less a Woman: Femininity, Sexuality & Breast Cancer.* New York: Hunter House Inc.

Kasper, A.S. (2000) Barriers and Burdens: Poor Women Face Breast Cancer. In Kasper, A.S. and Ferguson, S.J. (eds) *Breast Cancer: Society Shapes an Epidemic.* New York: St. Martin's Press.

Kaufert, P.A. (1998) Women, Resistance, and the Breast Cancer Movement. In Lock, M. and Kaufert, P.A. (eds) *Pragmatic Women and Body Politics.* New York: Cambridge University Press.

King, S. (2001) An all-consuming cause: breast cancer, corporate philanthropy, and the market for generosity, *Social Text*, 19, 4, 115–43.

Klawiter, M. (1999a) Racing for the cure, walking women, and toxic touring: mapping cultures of action within the Bay Area terrain of breast cancer, *Social Problems*, 46, 1, 104–26.

Klawiter, M. (1999b) Reshaping the Contours of Breast Cancer: From Private Stigma to Public Actions. Ph.D. Dissertation, Department of Sociology, University of California, Berkeley.

Klawiter, M. (2000) From Private Stigma to Global Assembly: Transforming the Terrain of Breast Cancer. In Burawoy, M., Blum, J., George, S., Gille, Z., Gowan, T., Haney, L., Klawiter, M., Lopez, S., O Riain, S. and Thayer, M. (eds) *Global Ethnography: Forces, Connections, and Imagination in a Postmodern World.* Berkeley, CA: University of California Press.

Klawiter, M. (2003) Chemicals, Cancer, and Prevention: The Synergy of Synthetic Social Movements. In Casper, M. (ed) *Synthetic Planet: Chemical Politics and the Hazards of Modern Life.* New York: Routledge.

Kleinman, A. (1988) *The Illness Narrative: Suffering, Healing and the Human Condition.* New York: Basic Books.

Kushner, R. (1975) *Breast Cancer: A Personal History and an Investigative Report.* New York: Harcourt Brace Jovanovich.

Kushner, R. (1977a) The Politics of Breast Cancer. In Dreifus, C. (ed) *Seizing Our Bodies: The Politics of Women's Health.* New York: Vintage.

Kushner, R. (1977b) *Why Me?: What Every Woman Should Know About Breast Cancer.* New York: New American Library.

Kushner, R. (1986) *Alternatives: New Developments in the War on Breast Cancer (with a new Introduction).* New York: Warner Books.

Lantz, P.M. and Booth, K.M. (1998) The social construction of the breast cancer epidemic, *Social Science and Medicine,* 46, 907–18.

Lantz, P.M., Weisman, C.S. and Itani, Z. (2003) A disease-specific Medicaid expansion for women: The Breast and Cervical Cancer Prevention and Treatment Act of 2000, *Women's Health Issues,* 13, 79–92.

Lawton, J. (2003) Lay experiences of health and illness: past research and future agendas, *Sociology of Health and Illness,* 25, Silver Anniversary Issue, 23–40.

Leopold, E. (1999) *A Darker Ribbon: Breast Cancer, Women, and Their Doctors in the Twentieth Century.* Boston, Massachusetts: Beacon Press.

Lerner, B.H. (2000) Inventing a Curable Disease: Historical Perspectives on Breast Cancer. In Ferguson, S.J. and Kasper, A.S. (eds) *Breast Cancer: The Social Construction of Illness.* New York: St. Martin's Press.

Lerner, B.H. (2001) *The Breast Cancer Wars: Hope, Fear, and the Pursuit of a Cure in Twentieth-Century America.* Oxford, England: Oxford University Press.

Linden, R.R. (1998) Writing the breast: screening mammography's contested history, 1976–1997, *Annual Meeting of the American Sociological Association,* San Francisco, CA.

Lorber, J. (1997) *Gender and the Social Construction of Illness.* Thousand Oaks: Sage.

Lorber, J. (1994) *Paradoxes of Gender.* New Haven: Yale University Press.

Lorde, A. (1980) *The Cancer Journals.* San Francisco: Aunt Lute books.

Love, S.M. with Lindsey, K. (1995) *Dr. Susan Love's Breast Book* (2nd edition). New York: Addison Wesley.

Lupton, D. (1995) *The Imperative of Health: Public Health and the Regulated Body.* Thousand Oaks, CA: Sage Publications, Inc.

Marino, C. and Gerlach, K.K. (1999) An analysis of breast cancer coverage in selected women's magazines, 1987–1995, *American Journal of Health Promotion,* 13, 3, 163–70.

Markle, G.E., Petersen, J.C. and Wagenfeld, M.O. (1978) Notes from the cancer underground: participation in the Laetrile Movement, *Social Science and Medicine,* 12, 31–7.

Mathews, H.F., Lannin, D.R. and Mitchell, J.P. (1994) Coming to terms with advanced breast cancer: black women's narratives from Eastern North Carolina, *Social Science and Medicine,* 38, 789–800.

Mayer, M. (1993) *Examining Myself: One Woman's Story of Breast Cancer Treatment and Recovery.* Boston: Faber & Faber.

McCormick, S., Brown, P. and Zavestoski, S. (2003) The personal is scientific, the scientific is political: the environmental breast cancer movement, *Sociological Forum,* 18, 4, 545–76.

Middlebrook, C. (1997) *Seeing the Crab.* New York: Doubleday.

Montini, T. (1996) Gender and emotion in the advocacy of breast cancer informed consent legislation, *Gender and Society,* 10, 1, 9–23.

Montini, T. (1997) Resist and redirect: physicians respond to breast cancer informed consent legislation, *Women and Health*, 26, 1, 85–105.

Montini, T. and Ruzek, S. (1989) Overturning orthodoxy: the emergence of breast cancer treatment policy, *Research in the Sociology of Health Care*, 8, 3–32.

Montini, T. and Slobin, K. (1991) Tensions between good science and good practice: lagging behind and leapfrogging ahead along the cancer care continuum, *Research in the Sociology of Health Care*, 9, 127–40.

Naples, N. (1998) *Community Activism and Feminist Politics: Organizing Across Race, Class, and Gender*. New York: Routledge.

National Institutes of Health (1979) *The Treatment of Primary Breast Cancer Management of Local Disease*. NIH Consensus Statement Online, 2, 5, 29–30. http://consensus.nih.gov/cons/015/015.intro.htm (last accessed 5 May 2004).

Norsigian, J. (1996) The Women's Health Movement in the United States. In Moss, K. (ed) *Man-Made Medicine: Women's Health, Public Policy and Reform*. Durham, NC: Duke University Press.

Olsen, O. and Gotzsche, P.C. (2001) Cochrane Review of screening for breast cancer with mammography, *The Lancet*, 358, 1340–42.

Orenstein, P. (1997) Breast cancer at 35: a diary of youth and loss, *New York Times Magazine*, Section 6.

Orenstein, S. (2003) The selling of breast cancer: is corporate america's love affair with a disease that kills 40,000 women a year good marketing – or bad medicine', *Busines2.0*, February.

Patterson, J.T. (1987) *The Dread Disease: Cancer and Modern American Culture*. Cambridge, MA: Harvard University Press.

Petersen, A. (1997) Risk, governance and the new public health. In Petersen, A. and Bunton, R. (eds) *Foucault, Health and Medicine*. New York: Routledge.

Petersen, A. and Bunton, R. (1997) *Foucault, Health and Medicine*. New York: Routledge.

Petersen, A. and Lupton, D. (1996) *The New Public Health: Health and Self in the Age of Risk*. Thousand Oaks, CA: Sage.

Pierret, J. (2003) The illness experience: state of knowledge and perspectives for research, *Sociology of Health and Illness*, 25, Silver Anniversary, 4–22.

Porter, R. (1985) The patient's view: doing history from below, *Theory and Society*, 14, 175–98.

Potts, L. (2000) Publishing the Personal: Autobiographical Narratives of Breast Cancer and the Self. In Potts, L. (ed) *Ideologies of Breast Cancer: Feminist Perspectives*. New York: St. Martin's Press.

Ray, R. (1998) Women's movements and political fields: a comparison of two Indian cities, *Social Problems*, 45, 1, 21–36.

Ray, R. (1999) *Fields of Protest: Women's Movements in India*. Minneapolis: University of Minnesota.

Rennie, S. (1977) Mammography: X-rated film, *Chrysalis*, 5, 21–33.

Rollin, B. (1976) *First You Cry*. New York: J.B. Lippincott.

Rosenbaum, M.E. and Roos, G.M. (2000) Women's Experiences of Breast Cancer. In Kasper, A.S. and Ferguson, S.J. (eds) *Breast Cancer: Society Shapes an Epidemic*. New York: St. Martin's Press.

Ross, W.S. (1987) *Crusade: The Official History of the American Cancer Society*. New York: Arbor House.

Ruzek, S.B. (1978) *The Women's Health Movement: Feminist Alternatives to Medical Control*. New York: Praeger.

Ruzek, S.B. and Becker, J. (1999) The women's health movement in the united states: from grass-roots activism to professional agendas, *Journal of the American Medical Women's Association (JAMWA)*, 54, 1, 4–9.

Saywell, C., Herderson, L. and Beattie, L. (2000) Sexualised Illness: the Newsworthy Body in Media Representations of Breast Cancer. In Potts, L. (ed) *Ideologies of Breast Cancer: Feminist Perspectives*. New York: St. Martin's Press.

Schaffer, E.R. (2000) Breast Cancer and the Evolving Health Care System: Why Health Care Reform Is a Breast Cancer Issue. In Kasper, A.S. and Ferguson, S.J. (eds) *Breast Cancer: Society Shapes an Epidemic*. New York: St. Martin's Press.

Scott, R.W., Ruef, M., Mendel, P.J. and Caronna, C.A. (2000) *Institutional Change and Healthcare Organizations: From Professional Dominance to Managed Care*. Chicago: University of Chicago.

Sherman, M. (2002) Doubts on mammograms do not affect their use, *New York Times*, 23rd June (electronic version).

Stein, R. (2004) Some fear women lack facts about mammograms, *Washington Post*, 6th January (electronic version).

Skrabanek, P. (1985) False premises and false promises of breast cancer screening, *The Lancet*, 10 August, 316–20.

Stocker, M. (1991) *Cancer As A Women's Issue: Scratching the Surface*. Chicago: Third Side Press.

Stocker, M. (1993) *Confronting Cancer, Constructing Change: New Perspectives on Women and Cancer*. Chicago: Third Side Press.

Strax, P., Venet, L. and Shapiro, S. (1973) Value of mammography in reduction of mortality from breast cancer in mass screening, *American Journal of Roentgenology*, 117, 3, 668–89.

Swissler, M.A. (2002) The Marketing of Breast Cancer, AlterNet.org 2002 (16th September).

Taylor, V. (1999) Gender and social movements: gender processes in women's self-help movements, *Gender and Society*, 13, 1, 8–33.

Taylor, V. and Van Willigen, M. (1996) Women's self-help and the reconstruction of gender: the postpartum support and breast cancer movements, *Mobilization: An International Journal*, 1, 2, 123–43.

Weisman, C.S. (2000) Breast Cancer Policymaking. In Kasper, A.S. and Ferguson, S.J. (eds) *Breast Cancer: Society Shapes an Epidemic*. New York, NY: St. Martins Press.

Winnow, J. (1989) Lesbians working on AIDS: assessing the impact on health care for women, *Out/Look*, 2 (Summer), 1, 10–18.

Winnow, J. (1991) Lesbians Evolving Health Care: Cancer and AIDS. In Brady, J. (ed) *1 in 3: Women with Cancer Confront an Epidemic*. San Francisco: Cleis Press.

Yadlon, S. (1997) Skinny women and good mothers: the rhetoric of risk, control, and culpability in the production of knowledge about breast cancer, *Feminist Studies*, 23, 3, 645–77.

Yalom, M. (1997) *A History of the Breast*. New York: Alfred A. Knopf.

Young, I.M. (1990) Breasted Experience: The Look and the Feel. In Young, I.M. (ed) *Throwing Like A Girl and Other Essays in Feminist Philosophy and Social Theory*. Bloomington, IN: Indiana University Press.

Zavestoski, S., Brown, P. and McCormick, S. (in press) Gendered bodies and disease: environmental breast cancer activists' challenges to science, the biomedical model, and policy, *Science as Culture*.

Index